THE BEST OF
NURSING HUMOR

THE BEST OF
NURSING HUMOR

A collection of
articles, essays,
and poetry
published in the
nursing literature

COMPILED AND EDITED BY

COLLEEN KENEFICK

ASSOCIATE LIBRARIAN, HEALTH SCIENCES LIBRARY
STATE UNIVERSITY OF NEW YORK AT STONY BROOK
STONY BROOK, NEW YORK

AMY Y. YOUNG

TECHNICAL SERVICES LIBRARIAN, HEALTH SCIENCES LIBRARY
STATE UNIVERSITY OF NEW YORK AT STONY BROOK
STONY BROOK, NEW YORK

HANLEY & BELFUS, Inc.
PHILADELPHIA

Publisher: HANLEY & BELFUS
210 S. 13th Street
Philadelphia, PA 19107
215-546-7293
Fax 215-790-9330

North American and worldwide sales and distribution:

MOSBY-YEAR BOOK, INC.
11830 Westline Industrial Drive
St. Louis, MO 63146

In Canada: MOSBY-YEAR BOOK, INC.
5240 Finch Avenue East
Unit 1
Scarborough, Ontario M1S 5A2
Canada

The Best of Nursing Humor   ISBN 1-56053-062-6

Library of Congress Catalog Card Number 92-75985

Last digit is the print number: 9 8 7 6 5 4 3 2

To Mom, Dad, Bonnie, and Sujato,
who tried to teach me not to sweat the big stuff.
To Grandpa Steffen,
who said it never rains at the beach,
it only comes off the trees.

CK

For Mom, Ken, and Scott,
who have, in their individual ways,
exemplified love, strength, and inspiration
in my wondrous journey through life.

AYY

CONTENTS

Acknowledgments   xi

Introduction   xiii

LEARNING THE HARD WAY

Survival Techniques . . . 3
BETTY BEAGLE, S.N.

The Student Nurse Slugging Syndrome . . . 4
RACHEL KENT AND KERRY ENSOLL

Some Days Are Like That! . . . 5
ROY BLAIR, R.N.

Good Nursing Practice (experimental
multiple choice exam theme) . . . 7
RADICAL NURSES GROUP

Good to the Last Drop . . . 8
ROY BLAIR, R.N.

Somewhere in the Land
of Curriculum Revision . . . 10
GAIL SCHOEN LeMAIRE, R.N., M.S.N.

The Voice . . . 11
ROY BLAIR, R.N.

Down the Tubes . . . 13
ETHEL GILLETTE, R.N., B.A.

Celebrity Musings . . . 15
LAURIE EYNON

Physiology Exam . . . 15
CARRIE HENGESBACH

Final Exams! . . . 16
SHIRLEY J. BRAVERMAN, R.N.

How Not to Pass Your Exams . . . 17
KEN CORK

Nursing School Days—Farewell . . . 19
CAROL WEIL, R.N.

Graduation Day . . . 20
PAMELA F. RICHTER, R.N.

The Board Game . . . 21
CONNIE MILNER, R.N.P.

IT'S NOT AS EASY AS IT LOOKS

A Nurse's Guide to Recruitment Ads . . . 25
JILL CURRY, R.N., B.A., C.E.N.

What the Ads Really Mean . . . 27

How to Read the Job Ads . . . 27

A Nurse Can Be a Man or a Woman . . . 28
ROSS P. MAYO

Of Caps and Shoes . . . 31
DELAILAH KHAN, R.N., B.Sc.N.

Transparent Benefits . . . 32
JILL L. CURRY, R.N., B.S.N., C.E.N.

E.D. Gazette . . . 34
SUSAN MOORE, R.N., B.S.N., C.C.R.N., C.E.N.

It Still Makes Me Cringe . . . 36
NEAL BUCKLEY, S.R.N., R.M.N.

How to Survive a Building Project . . . 37
ELLEN GORE, R.N., B.S.N.

The Olympic Athletes of Mill Town
Memorial . . . 40
ANNETTE RHODES, R.N., B.S.

Twenty-Two Laws They Wouldn't
Dare Enforce . . . 42
ROBERT W. PELTON

ANATOMY AND DIAGNOSIS

Medical Terminology for the Layman . . . 47

A Cilia Tale There Is Yet to Tell . . . 47
JENNY ASHMORE, PAUL GARDNER,
AND KAREN WALKER

"See If They Are A Live" . . . 49
KAREN M. JORDAN, C.O.R.T.

Anatomically Speaking . . . 50
ETHEL GILLETTE, R.N., B.A.

Why Do I Always Misdiagnose
the Patient I Know Best? . . . 51
SANDE JONES, R.N., M.S.

The Brotherhood of Motherhood . . . 53
SUSAN MOORE, R.N., B.S.N., C.C.R.N., C.E.N.

Diagnosing the Cat . . . 54
LINDA M. NORLANDER, R.N., B.S.N.

Bon Voyage? . . . 55
ANDREA KOVALESKY, R.N., M.S.N.

The Tale of the Innominate War . . . 56
SCOTT WRAIGHT

Twas the Night Before Christmas
(at PRN General) . . . 57
NANCY CORR, R.N., et. al.

NURSES VS. DOCTORS

How to Drive Nurses Crazy (and ease
them out of nursing) . . . 61
HARVEY N. MANDELL, M.D.

Spare the Fools and Interns . . . 63
THOM SCHWARZ, R.N.

Gown Tiers I Have Known . . . 65
B. S. CRAWFORD, M.B., F.R.C.S.

Gown Wearers I Have Known . . . 66
F. WHEELER, S.R.N.

Humor in the OR . . . 68
JOEL H. GOLDBERG

So You Want to Work in the OR . . . 69
KAREN M. JORDAN, C.S.T.

Communicating with Surgeons,
Once You Learn the Language,
Is Possible Most of the Time . . . 71
PATTY SWENSON, R.N.

WATCH YOUR LANGUAGE

Acute, Fulminating Jargonitis . . . 75
ELLEN GOLDENSOHN

Nurses, Nuances, and Non-Communication:
A Humorous Look at Language . . . 76
RICHARD M. GRIMES, PhD AND
RONALD J. LORIMOR, PhD

"The Password, Please" . . . 78
SUSAN MOORE, R.N., B.S.N., C.C.R.N., C.E.N.

How to Present a Mortality
and Morbidity Conference . . . 79
IRVING L. KRON, M.D.

How Well Do You Communicate? . . . 80
MANCHESTER RADICAL NURSES GROUP

How the *Write* Stuff
Can Go Wrong . . . 81
AVICE H. KERR, R.N., B.A.

Charting Chuckles . . . 84
BARBARA WYAND WALKER, R.N., B.S.N.

This Is What the Doctor Dictated . . . 85
PETER GOTT, M.D.

Raw Data . . . 86
ROBERT S. HOFFMAN, M.D.

The Nunsuch Handbook . . . 88
RONALD J. MIHORDIN

Bedpan Blues . . . 90
STEVEN TIGER

Comments Nurses Could Live Without . . . 91
VIRGINIA MOORE DEWEES, R.N.

WHERE ARE WE?

Origins of Nursing Knowledge . . . 95
MARY R. INGRAM, R.N., M.S.

Can You See Me? . . . 96
MICHAEL A. CARTER, D.N.S.c., R.N., F.A.A.N.

"In-Basket" Research:
An Education for Educators . . . 97
LAUREL ARCHER COPP, PH.D., R.N., F.A.A.N.

Invasion of the Busybodies . . . 99
ANGELA PLUME

Nurses: Playgirls on the Boob Tube? . . . 100
LEAH L. CURTIN, R.N.

Leadership Styles . . . 102
JOAN M. WABSCHALL

On Milking Sacred Cows . . . 103
LEAH L. CURTIN, R.N.

I Want To Be a Soap Opera Nurse . . . 105
VIRGINIA MOORE DEWEES, R.N.

TV Nurses: Sexy, Deferential—
and Phony . . . 106
ARLENE ORHON JECH, R.N.

Nurse Manners' Guide
to Politically Correct Behavior . . . 107
ANGELA E. VINCENZI, R.N., ED.D.

Mother Goose *Nursing* Rhymes
by Mother Goose . . . 109
GLORIA ROSENTHAL

PATIENTS AND OTHER STRANGERS

Sex in the Hospital . . . 113
LEAH L. CURTIN, R.N.

"You Swallowed Your WHAT!" . . . 115
JANE THOMPSON DOYLE, R.N., B.S.N.

Take a Big Breath, Hold It,
And . . . Burst Out Laughing . . . 117
JOAN PERRY, R.N.

Take Time to Laugh . . . 118
CATHLEEN HUCKABY, R.N.

Medical Education Upgraded . . . 119
G. K. STANTON

Hip Remarks . . . 120
ROY B. MOORE

Who Says Being an ICU Patient Is No Fun? . . . 121
WILLIAM J. RYAN, M.D.

No Peace in Hospital . . . 123
JOAN JARVIS

The Other Side of the Sheets . . . 124
LES DAWSON

Angels of Mercy . . . 125
SANDRA L. WREN, B.A.

REALITY 101

How to Assess Your Unit
Before You Take Report . . . 129
NANCY ARMSTRONG

Job Description for Nursing Supervisor:
The Unwritten Realities . . . 130
JUDITH K. PARKER

On Games People Play in Hospitals . . . 131
THELMA M. LANKFORD, R.N.

Reality Testing . . . 132
CAROL E. CLELAND, R.N., B.S.

Listen Here! . . . 133
VIRGINIA MOORE DeWEES, R.N.

What They Don't Teach You
in Nursing School . . . 134
SUZANNE GOLIGHTLY, R.N., B.S.N.

Things Our Instructors Never Told Us . . . 135
KATHLEEN POOLE, R.N., B.S.N.

Hospital Equipment . . . 136
ROY BLAIR, R.N.

Elevator Excursions . . . 139
TANYA M. SUDIA ROBINSON, M.N., R.N.

Telesco's Laws . . . 140
MARIA TELESCO

If Oliver North Taught
Hospital Administration . . . 141
MARY B. MALLISON, R.N.

AS TIME GOES BY

Hickory Dickory . . . A Fable
for Our Times . . . 145
JOAN M. RINEHART, R.N., PH.D.

Bandwagons Nursing Has Jumped On—
or Off: A Satire on Some of the Events
in the History of Nursing Education . . . 146
MARION M. SCHRUM, ED.D., R.N.

I'm an Upwardly Mobile Stick-in-the-Mud . . . 149
GILLESPIE RICHARDS, R.N., B.A.

I Never Wear White After Dark . . . 150
PAULINE J. ALLEY, L.P.N.

My Love Affair with Uniforms . . . 151
MARY JANE JANOWSKI, R.N., B.S.N.

The More Things Change . . . 153
EDITH P. LEWIS, R.N., M.N., F.A.A.N.

Why I'm Superstitious
About Nurse's Curses . . . 154
GRETCHEN COURTRIGHT, R.N.

If You're Married to a Nurse . . . 155
GILLESPIE RICHARDS, R.N., B.A.

Hazardous (to the) Waist . . . 156
TED ROBERTS

The Good, the Bad, and the Ugly . . . 158
DONNA HARRISON STAAB, M.S.N., B.S.N., R.N.

Going Over the Hill . . . 159
CATHERINE M. NORRIS, R.N.

The Last Nurse . . . 161
MELODY ALLISON, R.N., B.S.N.

Author Index . . . 163

Bibliography . . . 165

ACKNOWLEDGMENTS

This volume represents the combined talents of many individuals whose excellent pieces have made our editorial task easy.

We wish to convey special thanks to Jerry Fisch and Ruth Marcolina.

We owe a particular debt to Brian Epp, illustrator of the volume, for his skill and forbearance.

We gratefully acknowledge the able and patient assistance, unstinting enthusiasm, and support of our editor Linda Belfus and her staff at Hanley and Belfus.

To the many individuals who have given so generously of their time and expertise in the course of preparation of this book, we wish to extend our sincere gratitude.

INTRODUCTION

A couple of years ago right before the end of fall semester, when the library was almost deserted, we overheard two nursing students complain about their classes and their interminable reading lists. We smiled at the familiar comments, but something struck a nerve when we heard one of them say "and none of it is even funny!"

Being medical librarians and having quirky senses of humor, we decided to find out for ourselves if there was any validity to that statement. Unable to locate material in a single volume on the topic of nursing humor, we began by searching Medline, CINAHL and the Nursing Studies Index. Most of the material in these indexes were articles about using humor as a coping mechanism or as a teaching tool. After a preliminary search, we were ready to agree that there really was nothing funny in the nursing literature.

Undaunted by the paucity of material, we decided to examine recent journals more carefully. An explosive growth in nursing journals occurred in the 1970s and, with this in mind, we decided to start with 1970 and end with June 1992. Eventually we spent untold hours scanning cover to cover 60 some journals published between 1970 and 1992. It became difficult to locate humorous pieces in most of the leading nursing journals published since the mid 1980s. Journals that had previous published humor or satire had eliminated those sections. Only North American and British journals were perused, with 33 journals eventually being represented in this collection. Our original intention was to select material only from nursing journals, but the search led us to pieces that were too good not to be included.

The following guidelines governed our selection process. All of the material had to be written by or about nurses. Every article had to say something about at least one aspect of the nursing profession and it had to make us laugh, chuckle, or at least smile. Humor comes in various styles, and since we both have very different senses of humor, we decided that we had to agree on the inclusion of each and every piece. We made no attempt to exclude material that may be viewed as sexist or controversial; rather the goal was to have a representative sample. Every effort was made to explore the rich diversity of nursing life. If more than one article covered the same subject, we included the funniest one or the one that we thought would have the broadest appeal. Some chapters are longer than others because more published material was found in those areas. Many of the articles selected deal with interrelationships and communication between colleagues, families, and patients, in keeping with the current emphasis on the humanistic side of medicine and nursing.

To authors and readers whose favorite material is not included, we apologize for the oversight. Please send us your cherished selections so that they can be reviewed for the next edition.

The articles are divided into nine chapters that chronicle the stages a typical nurse experiences during the course of a long career. Beginning with the trials and tribulations of nursing school, neophytes then discover the perils of job hunting. At this juncture, they also receive the first glimpse of "real-life" nursing. In the third chapter, the new nurse learns to cope with a plethora of diseases along with the nuts and bolts of treatment regimens. Learning to cooperate with physicians and using communication effectively are of paramount importance in a nurse's daily work. The sixth chapter details the world of academics and the mass media's perceptions of the nursing profession. With courage, humility, and compassion, the wonderful world of patient care is depicted. Exposing the realities of day-to-day nursing is the essence of chapter eight. In the final chapter, the fulfillment of pursuing this role over time is examined.

An extensive bibliography is included because many excellent articles were omitted. Most of these articles are of the same quality as those that were selected but did not fit into one of the nine chapters. Also, when both editors could not agree on the merits of a piece, it was excluded but listed in the bibliography. Unfortunately, many outstanding articles are included in the bibliography because copyright permission could not be obtained.

We hope that this volume will appeal to nurses, their families, and their associates in other health-care professions. Not every article will appeal to every reader, but everyone should find something entertaining within these pages. So sit back, put your feet up, relax, and enjoy.

Colleen Kenefick
Amy Y. Young

LEARNING THE HARD WAY

Angels of mercy are made, not born. They begin earning their wings each and every day in nursing school. These awestruck neophytes face a pathway fraught with anxiety and confusion, and their learning can be slow and disappointing.

Nursing students must possess a ready wit and an uncanny ability to interact with people from diverse backgrounds. Fortunately, with good common sense and hard work, these fledgling angels are molded into efficient, competent professionals ready to fly on their own.

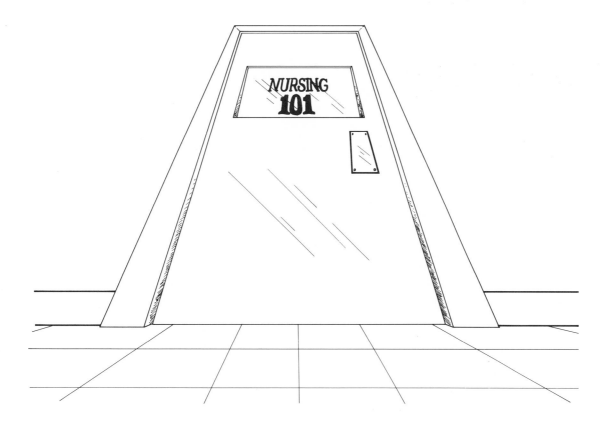

Survival Techniques*

BETTY BEAGLE, S.N.

You finally did it, you have decided nursing is what you want to do for the rest of your life. After all, who would go through all this anguish if you only wanted to do this as a pastime? If you are taking this like everyone else, you are probably going to do this by trial and error, "war" stories, or by helpful hints from the nursing staff.

You need to prioritize your time. This is a familiar and much used term which you will hear often. It is also easier said than done!

If you are single, you have an advantage—maybe. You can decide right now that single is "where it's at" and stay that way for the duration. Of course this means literally living the "single" life. There are no "dinners-for-two," no telephone conversations, no movies at the cinema (rarely any TV), in other words no physical contact with the opposite sex. I know you weren't thinking about it anyway but in case you are studying anatomy and physiology and hormonal thoughts pervade your consciousness, dismiss them.

If you are married, I am not suggesting divorce, just abstinence. Hopefully, you kissed your spouse goodbye when you came to school for your first day of class because your next chance will be on your breaks or when you graduate.

If you happen to be a parent, do as I did. I put pictures of myself in all rooms of my house when I started to school so my kids wouldn't forget me. My children, in return, helped me by plastering their faces on my fridge (they know I'll look there) or on my mirror (another sure spot).

I have acquired a son-in-law, a daughter-in-law, and five grandchildren in the past two and a half years and I usually don't recognize them if I run into them on the rare occasions when I go to the store for essentials (like food) or out to pay our utility bills. Christmas is fun though, because each year I get to spend a few days getting to know the family again. But we all must wear name tags for the first day!

If your children are small, buy them the Fisher Price Kitchen and teach them how to "cook" nourishing "hot" cereal on the stove that doesn't heat up. For the infant, hang a TPN (hint: Total *Parental* Nutrition) of Similac with iron at 40 cc/hr that the baby can control by sound! Crying should do it! Instead of a needle, use a nipple . . .

Diapers—what would we do without those disposable diapers that stay dry for two weeks at a time? You can even buy the kind that you touch the waist band and Mickey Mouse and his friends jump off to entertain your baby.

Some of you may feel guilty about not fixing those delicious meals your family once enjoyed. Don't! We get two "breaks" a year and during that time fix barrels of nourishing liquid (you can add a few veggies) and when your family gets hungry, just take out enough to keep fluids and lytes balanced. Remind them that this is only going to last another year or two.

Have I covered everything? Oh, I forgot dust . . . Dust used to bother me, but not anymore. I use it to write notes to my 17 year old, to let him know what time I am going to be in the house so he won't mistake me for a burglar, and to say *I Love You.*

On a serious note, each semester you will get regrouped with new classmates. They will become your family, your support group. You will form a chain and everyone is a strong link. This is a group effort. These are people who will laugh with you and cry with you. You will form friendships that will last a lifetime. Take advantage of these opportunities.

On a closing note—do not listen to all the "war stories" that go around—just to the credible ones . . . like mine!

---

*Reprinted from Advancing Clinical Care, ©1990; 5(3):17 with permission from Data Design, Inc., Franksville, Wisconsin.

The Student Nurse Slugging Syndrome*

RACHEL KENT
KERRY ENSOLL

1. **A student nurse shows her initiative**
Would you:
(a) Panic
(b) Reprimand her and tell her not to do it again
(c) Refer her for a brain scan
(d) Lay her down in the rest room for a few hours

2. **A student nurse speaks directly to a visiting consultant**
Would you:
(a) Resuscitate the consultant
(b) Intubate the offending nurse thus preventing any recurrence of verbal communication
(c) Lock her in the nursing officer's compartment for a few days

3. **A student nurse is found letting a drip run too fast**
Would you tell her:
(a) The doctors are not here to be exhausted
(b) The Techmar is not an adding machine
(c) To wipe her nose

4. **A student nurse is found maliciously attacking the ITU technician with a stretcher pole**
Would you:
(a) Help her
(b) Take a blood sample for gas analysis
(c) Remove his spectacles and/or dentures, lest they become damaged during the procedure

5. **A student nurse is exposed while an X-ray is being taken**
Would you:
(a) Tell her to put her uniform back on
(b) Send her for fertility tests
(c) Console her and say it's always an advantage to have experience in blue movies

6. **A student nurse is learning about cardiac monitoring**
Would you instruct her that:
(a) A straight line does not always mean the vertical hold is up the chute!
(b) If she fiddles with the controls she can pick up "Top of the Pops" on bed three
(c) Brady Cardia is a good friend of yours and can't help being a bit slow!

7. **A student nurse begins to act strangely in the unit**
Would you think:
(a) This is obviously a side-effect of being an earthworm!
(b) She must have kicked the glue-sniffing and started on Cidex!
(c) You wish she'd stop imitating the trained staff

8. **A student nurse reports to you the discovery of a staff nurse and anaesthetist ensconced in Room 1**
Would you:
(a) Run to join in
(b) Tell her to observe as it would be a good learning experience
(c) Turn the temperature control down to cool their ardor

9. **A student nurse is taught about the use of an airbed**
Would you tell her:
(a) ITU is not an appropriate place for trampoline practice
(b) She need not have used a bicycle pump to inflate it!
(c) She was not supposed to test it with the houseman

10. **When compiling the final reports of the present student nurses**
Should you:
(a) Try not to give them too many As
(b) Ensure that you've had at least four pints of Guinness before starting
(c) Find out from the domestic who they were anyway!

* Reprinted from Nursing Times, ©1984; 80(26):46 with permission from Macmillan Magazines, Ltd.

Some Days Are Like That!*

ROY BLAIR, R.N.

"I always have the students stand here," the head nurse said, indicating an area about the size of a telephone booth. The ten of us obediently crammed ourselves in. It was the first day on the surgical ward and we were gathered at the desk for report. Our instructor made shooing motions, trying to push us even farther out of the way.

The policy on this ward concerning reports seemed to be that they were classified information and as students we didn't have the proper clearance; we were placed as far away from them as possible.

"Why don't they just put us in the linen closet and shut the door," somebody behind me muttered.

Following the inaudible night report, our clinical instructor said, "I would like to see your nursing care plans." This was the part I dreaded most.

Our instructor made us write long, elaborate and detailed nursing care plans. Everything that was done for the patient, every move we made had to be written down and justified. When we were given a new patient assignment, we prepared a care plan that made the Royal Wedding look like an impulse.

My written work always came back covered with so many red slashes that I thought it had been marked by Zorro. However, the day I wrote that the patient's low back pain was due to a lumpy mattress, one of my instructor's wheels slipped a cog.

"I don't know why you are having so much trouble," she said, "any idiot can write a nursing care plan. Why, I've done hundreds of them myself."

I wasn't about to argue with that statement. I handed her my care plans which she read quickly, shaking her head.

"Your patient in room six is having a hernia repair this morning, so he requires a shave prep," she stated.

Great, I thought sarcastically, this is a first for me and with my luck he'll have more hair on him than King Kong.

We entered the utility room.

"How long will it take you to do this procedure?" my instructor asked.

Well, I thought, taking into consideration skin grafts, suturing and transfusions, about two weeks.

Out loud I said, "twenty minutes."

"Get your equipment."

I went around the loaded shelves and picked out about one of everything I could find.

She surveyed the untidy heap on the counter and asked sardonically, "What else do you think you'll need.?"

"A get-away car," I ventured.

She gave me a look that placed me high on her endangered species list. I gathered everything up and we proceeded to the patient's room, me dropping odds and ends of equipment along the corridor as if I were blazing a trail.

"You go in first," she said.

"Why?" I asked, "isn't he friendly? Should I duck?"

"Go in and introduce yourself," she sighed, "then explain what you are going to do."

At this point, I couldn't even remember my own name, so I just announced, "I have come to shave you." The patient rubbed his chin.

"No, the area where the doctor will be operating." I pointed vaguely at his sheet-covered body.

My instructor shook her head and left. I set up the equipment. The prep soap, true to form, was ice cold and the patient jumped a foot when I touched him. So did I. Then he noticed the shaking hand which held the razor and started to shake also. This seemed to set the tone for the entire event. He would jump, followed by my reflex movement and then we would both shake in unison.

I am happy to say that I got through the entire procedure without a scratch, and so did the patient. When I offered him a small curl of pubic hair for the family Bible, he accepted it with thankful relief.

* Reproduced with permission from The Canadian Nurse/L'infirmiere canadienne, ©1982; 78(10):46–47.

"Your next patient is due for surgery in one hour," my instructor announced, "go over the Operating Room check list with her." I took the list to the patient's room.

"Makeup removed?" I asked. She nodded.

"False teeth?"

"Yes, but may I keep them in until it's time to go?"

I gestured affirmatively. "Nail polish removed?" She nodded again.

"Glass eye?" I asked with a smile. She pointed to her left eye.

"Can I keep it until it's time to go?"

"Yes," I responded. I then glanced nervously at her hair.

"Wig?"

"Yes," she said, patting it in a friendly fashion, "but can I keep it till it's time to go?"

I nodded and then looked at the next item on the list and, with a trembling voice, asked, "artificial limbs?"

She threw back the covers and pointed to her right leg. I left the room to the tune of, "Can I keep it with me till it's time to go?" I had the vision of wheeling her to the O.R. in an untidy heap of disconnected parts, while forgetting the part that they were going to operate on.

"Have you ever removed a drain?" my instructor inquired. We were back in the utility room.

"No Ma'am," I replied, "I was always afraid of flooding the kitchen."

"A surgical drain," she continued, using that tone of voice that people reserve for backward children. "The patient in room three is to have her drain removed and dressing changed. I want you to do it; get whatever you need."

Our instructor's policy for these procedures was, "do it until you get it right." This usually produced one of three results: the patient fell asleep from sheer boredom, the student became hysterical or the instructor was institutionalized.

I had changed a dressing before and, remembering that I drop nearly everything I pick up, gathered a large supply of everything. We proceeded to the patient's room, my instructor leading the way. I followed, loaded down like a pack mule.

I explained the procedure to the patient and then opened the sterile packages, losing a number of dressings just for a start.

"Grasp the end of the drain with your forceps," my instructor said, "then pull gently."

Now, forceps and I just don't click. In my hands, their tips, like a committee, never get together on anything. After a number of false starts, though, I managed to get a grip on the slippery drain and pulled. Nothing happened.

"Pull a little harder," my instructor hissed at me.

Suddenly the drain started to move. Inch by inch it slipped out. I couldn't believe how long it was. Just as I was having visions of being out in the hall and still pulling, it let go. Unfortunately, so did I. It shot past my ear and with a light plopping sound hit the ceiling, where it stuck. We all stared up at it, and the patient started to giggle.

I worked my way through the rest of the procedure, following my custom of dropping every second thing I picked up. This was done to the accompaniment of the patient's hysterical laughter. Finally, as the dressings were piling up around my feet like small untidy snowdrifts, I applied the last piece of adhesive.

"I have never been entertained so much in years," the patient gasped, tears running down her cheeks. "If I had known it was going to be so funny, I would have invited my bridge club."

I returned to the utility room to clean up the tray.

"The patient you prepped this morning has returned from the O.R.," my instructor announced. "Tomorrow you can get him out of bed for the first time."

I stopped banging stainless steel equipment around the sink and thought, he stands six foot two and weighs 210 pounds. It should be a fun experience.

But that's another story.

Good Nursing Practice*
(experimental multiple choice exam theme)

RADICAL NURSES GROUP

1. Your off-duty has been changed while you were on your day off. Do you:
(a) Apologize profusely for causing so much trouble?
(b) Come in on your original shift?
(c) Go home?
(d) Work both the early and the late shift?

2. A patient decides to take her own discharge. Do you:
(a) Sit on her until the doctor arrives?
(b) Help pack her bags?
(c) Tranquillize her?
(d) Offer her reassurance, in a deep, soothing voice?

3. A patient asks for a glass of water on the doctor's round. Do you:
(a) Ignore him?
(b) Tell the doctor?
(c) Explain why it is physiologically unsound to drink?
(d) Make a note in the Kardex—"Patient attention seeking"?

4. A doctor tells you to get her stethoscope from the office. Do you:
(a) Run quickly, leaving a patient on a bedpan?
(b) Say, "Get it yourself" and vanish for the rest of the shift?
(c) Scowl darkly but get it anyway?
(d) Delegate the task to a junior nurse?

5. A nursing officer finds you talking to a patient. Do you:
(a) Thrust a thermometer into the patient's mouth?
(b) Apologize profusely?
(c) Run quickly in the opposite direction?
(d) Introduce the nursing officer by her first name?

6. You are found drinking tea in the kitchen by the SNO during your break. Do you:
(a) Apologize profusely?
(b) Thrust the cup into a patient's hand?
(c) Pour a second cup?
(d) Offer to work extra time?

7. Your shop steward comes to inform you of the next branch meeting. Do you:
(a) Say loudly, "Yes, I'd love to come to your party"?
(b) Walk straight past her and look the other way?
(c) Get her off the ward as quickly as possible?
(d) Call the security officer?

8. You are found by a Radical Nurse smiling at a doctor. Do you:
(a) Apologize profusely?
(b) Say apologetically, "He's all right really"?
(c) Start to ignore him?
(d) Say loudly, "How dare you underestimate my ability to make decisions"?

9. It's your first day on a new ward and you are asked to give a report. Do you:
(a) Say, "Good night—slept well" for each patient, and hope no one will notice?
(b) Pretend not to have heard?
(c) Faint quietly in the corner?
(d) Go off sick?

*Reprinted from Nursing Times, ©1983; 79(12):23 with permission from Macmillan Magazines, Ltd.

Good to the Last Drop*

ROY BLAIR, R.N.

"Don't get your medications ready too early," my instructor said. "They could get dusty."

I'll remember that, I thought. I have enough to do without dusting pills. This was my first experience with medications, and I was nervous.

We were in the tiny medicine room which was painted that depressing color known as Operating-Room-Green. A large bulletin board partly covered one wall. Among the old and faded messages was one signed F. Nightingale. A much newer notice, signed by the head nurse, was a request that, "When storing stool specimens in the fridge, do not put them on my lunch." I think somebody was trying to tell her something.

Most of the floor space in this little room was occupied by a quite large and very old fridge which spent its time rearranging its various internal parts into more comfortable positions. This task was accompanied by long Cheyne-Stokes rattles and loud congested nasal sighs. On damp days, it occasionally emitted a loud shriek, as if suddenly stabbed by a rheumatic pain. When that happened anyone who happened to be in the room jumped and dropped whatever they were holding.

"Here are your patient's medicine cards," my instructor said. "Get your medications ready."

I fumbled around in the cupboard and, finally locating the proper bottle, read the label carefully and removed the cap. Then I attempted to jiggle one pill out of the bottle and into the upturned cap. Three dropped out. I up-ended the cap and all three scooted back into the bottle. On the second try, I got four out and put four back. On the third try, I managed one-half a pill and returned it. I looked into the bottle. There they were—about 30 small, round, defiant objects. The scored line across the center gave the appearance of a tight, stubborn little mouth on a flat, round face. I felt like inserting a finger and knocking them around a bit,

just to show who was boss. The pills, however, had the upper hand and they knew it.

I decided that a little self-assertion was necessary and gave the bottle an angry shake. Like children suddenly released from a classroom the majority of them flew out in every direction. They cartwheeled happily around the counter and finally hid themselves coyly under everything available. I rooted out as many as I could find, dropped one into the portion cup, and stuffed the rest back into the bottle.

The fridge chose this moment to rearrange its shelf contents, making as much noise as possible. My instructor remained ominously silent.

The next card called for half a pill. I looked into the bottle. There were about six half tablets, but no matter how often I shook them out, only whole ones appeared.

"Break one," my instructor said in a tired voice.

I hate trying to break a pill in half, as I always end up with a little pile of powder. I tried, however, with predictable results. I tried again. And again.

"How old is your patient?" my instructor inquired.
"Ninety-two."

"Perhaps," she said quietly, "you had better hurry."
I tried again—ditto.

"How many chances do you have left?" she asked.
I eyeballed the remaining contents of the bottle.
"About two dozen."

"Continue," she said in a tone of voice that suggested that if I had been suddenly zapped into outer space I wouldn't be missed.

The counter was littered with the broken bodies of my antagonists. I had created enough dust to land me with at least three counts of air pollution but I persisted. On the next try, I was partially successful. I managed to hold onto one half, while the other flew off in a southerly direction.

Both my instructor and the fridge sighed with relief.

* Reproduced with permission from The Canadian Nurse/L'infirmiere canadienne, ©1983; 79(3):45.

The next medication order was for two capsules. Now, tablets and capsules have distinctly different personalities. Tablets are individuals with few social abilities. Capsules, on the other hand, have a tendency to stick together like a bunch of teenagers and this cohesive ability can defy even the sharpest fingernail. I managed, with considerable difficulty, to pry two loose from the rest of the gang.

The last card called for a liquid. I picked up the bottle. In large letters was the instruction, "Shake Well Before Using."

"Always check the . . ." my instructor began, but my arm was already in motion. The cap flew off and a thick, bright orange liquid erupted from the top of the bottle like a miniature Mount St. Helen's. I closed my eyes.

". . . cap first," she concluded in a strained voice. I opened my eyes.

The touches of orange on the walls gave the room a rather festive air. My instructor's expression suggested that justifiable homicide should be included in the penal code, while behind me the fridge chuckled.

As a student nurse, I had been storing away some valuable bits of information. For instance "disposable" meant an object could not be recycled. (Rinse it out; we can use it for a vase.) "Portable" meant with a crane. Anything labelled "adjustable" required a hammer. To this list, I added, "shake well before using," which I now knew meant after checking the cap, and never in the vicinity of a clinical instructor.

We cleaned up the bright, sticky liquid as well as we could and I tried again. I poured the prescribed amount into the medicine glass, but one last drop clung to the lip of the bottle.

What followed is something I will never forget. The old saying, "good to the last drop" took on a whole new meaning.

I tilted the bottle slightly. The drop stretched down towards the medicine glass and then, just when I thought I was in the driver's seat, it retracted back to its original shape and position.

I tapped the bottle against the glass. I banged, squeezed, jarred and jolted it. I agitated and shook it. I did everything but lick it off. All to no avail.

"Are you becoming spastic?" my instructor inquired. She handed me a cloth and, defeated, I wiped the bottle and replaced the cap.

"Now take the tray, we'll go to the patient's room and, for heaven's sake, don't drop it." Whatever gave her that idea?

Together we trudged down the hall, two prematurely aged people dressed in white with sticky orange spots. By the way, it isn't difficult to dust a pill once you learn how to hang on to it.

Somewhere in the Land of Curriculum Revision*

GAIL SCHOEN LeMAIRE, R.N., M.S.N.

Once upon a time, a nursing faculty undertook the process of curriculum revision, beginning with the formulation of a philosophy and conceptual framework. The atmosphere during curriculum meetings was almost always emotionally charged. Arguments erupted concerning apparently trivial matters. Formerly amiable colleagues became arch enemies, at times secretly vowing to destroy each other while disagreements seethed. Sentences were rewritten time after time with an over-emphasis on the placement of semicolons, colons, and periods. Paragraphs were moved, altered, rewritten, bisected and disected, ad infinitum. Consensus was rarely reached concerning grammatical issues; discussion was usually accompanied by the pounding of fists and the slamming of doors. (A task which involved 12 people trying to write one sentence is insane!) On the other hand, one should question the sanity of those who seek to be involved in that task!

Nursing faculty know that the philosophy and conceptual framework are vital parts of the curriculum. Faculty also know that the development of these two items is a painful process which, although it may ultimately be satisfying, may also lead to frustration, annoyance and antagonism. Unless precautions are taken, the process of curriculum revision can become endless. It seems necessary then, for faculty to learn to revise curriculum in a constructive, healthy, and happy way. Below are some hopefully helpful hints and suggestions for "how to revise happily ever after."

Ten Ways to Survive Curriculum Revision and Live Happily Ever After

1. Sit next to a person who is not your best friend. (You're likely to whisper to one another about others, enabling you to become close and work together better.)

2. See that refreshments are available—even if you have to bring them. (Full stomachs engage in happier revision.)

3. Ensure that grammatical issues are addressed by one or two expert individuals. (A dozen people will never agree on the placement of a comma.)

4. If you feel the urge to strangle a colleague—take a walk; head toward the restroom. (Going to the bathroom will provide more satisfaction than committing murder.)

5. If you really don't know what a philosophy is—find out. (It's easier to write something if you know what it is.)

6. If you don't understand what a conceptual framework is, don't worry too much. (You soon will.)

7. If you doubt the importance of a philosophy and conceptual framework, learn to value them. (You cannot complete what you think is a worthless task.)

8. If you find that the process of revision is depressing, put a vase of flowers in the center of the table. (A cheerful environment will raise your spirits.)

9. If you find that the process has come to a standstill, change rooms. (Looking at new walls will increase the circulation to your brain, leading to fresh ideas.)

10. If you want the revision to be completed yesterday—slow down. (Neither Rome nor your curriculum will be built in a day!)

*Reprinted from Journal of Nursing Education, ©1985; 24(5):218 with permission from Slack, Inc.

The Voice*

ROY BLAIR, R.N.

"Don't stand around the halls," she roared. "It makes the place look untidy."

This was our first day as students in the operating room. After our classroom theory, administered by this instructor at the top of her lungs, one would think we would be used to her, but we weren't. Everybody jumped and ran in different directions. While most of my fellow students seemed to follow the flight plan of a deflating balloon, I couldn't move. I have never been able to react quickly after being startled, so I was easy prey.

"What are you doing?" she demanded in a voice that loosened the ceiling tiles.

"Nothing Ma'am," I stammered.

"Well, do something."

"Yes, Ma'am," I replied, making a quick left turn and running into the wall.

Our clinical instructor had been a military nurse. She brought to this civilian job a wealth of experience and dedication. She walked with a distinctive limp acquired, according to rumor, from falling off a camel during a tour of duty in Africa. Something else left over from her military days was a voice that could carry for blocks.

"The Voice," as we referred to her, struck terror into the hearts of students and graduate nurses as well. She was always on the alert for breaks in sterile technic. Nobody escaped her eagle eye. Even the surgeons were marched back to the scrub sink with orders to "Do it again and this time do it right."

She had one other very disturbing characteristic besides her voice. This was the ability to materialize at your elbow, even if you were just thinking about doing something you shouldn't. This sudden appearance was always accompanied by a roar that shrivelled your eardrum.

"If you touch that, I'll cut your hand off," seemed to be a favorite expression. I believed her!

On one Friday afternoon, she sent us on our way with the parting shot, "Learn the hemorrhoid setup and dirty case routine; and if you don't know it by Monday, don't come back."

It was now Monday morning and she had already caught us loitering in the OR corridor.

"Go to room nine and scrub for the hemorrhoid case," she ordered. I was the only student left, so I slunk away in the general direction of room nine.

I scrubbed my hands for the allotted time without incident and even managed the gown and gloves. Then I set up the table, placing the instruments together in neat, sociable little groups. The circulating nurse pushed a small table into the room, which she deposited near me, and then left again. On the table was a long silver cylindrical instrument with one tapered end. The other end had wires attached which ran down to a small brown box on the lower shelf of the table.

"What could that be used for," I thought nervously. Alone in the room, I leaned over for a closer look.

"Don't touch that," the Voice roared. I jumped as if I'd been stabbed.

"That table is not sterile," she declared. "You will be contaminated if you touch it."

Contaminated was a word feared by every student. I had visions of her hanging a sign around my neck which would read unclean.

"That is a sigmoidoscope," she stated. "Don't you know what a sigmoidoscope is used for?"

"No," I replied innocently. "What do you do with it?" For a moment she just stood there looking at me. Then she turned and left the room. Later when I found out what the instrument was used for, I had to admire her restraint.

At the end of the operation, I began the task of cleaning the instruments and equipment according to the routine procedure. This was done to the accompaniment of The Voice pointing out, in unnecessary detail, every mistake I made, including getting up that morning.

The last step of this routine was emptying the pail of dirty water into the hopper. She came with me to the

* Reprinted from Point of View, ©1984; 21(2):18–19, with permission from Ethicon, Inc.

utility room where I poured the contents of the pail into the hopper. She pressed the handle to flush it. There was a flash of silver and a metallic clink as the detachable, tapered end of the sigmoidoscope flowed out of the pail and into the hopper. We watched, fascinated, as it rolled with the current around the inside of the bowl, in ever decreasing circles. Then it disappeared down the drain.

"I suggest," she said sarcastically, "that during your nursery experience you check the bathwater carefully before you throw it out."

My first experience with a major case was as second scrub.

"You can gown and glove the doctors," the first scrub said. She should have known better.

I held out the glove for the surgeon. He drove his hand in so hard that the glove separated in half. The finger portion remained on his hand, while the cuff, which I still clung to, travelled up to his shoulder.

"How many years did you train to learn that?" he asked.

I was relegated to the back table for the rest of the operation. Here I spent my time fumbling with sponges on holders and tying suture into knots: two occupations for which I had a definite talent.

Sometimes a second scrub student was used to hold a retractor. On rare occasions, we were asked to cut suture. However, placing scissors in the hand of a nervous, shaking student nurse was akin to letting Jack the Ripper loose in the operating room. One surgeon said, as he retrieved the scissors, "I make the incisions, nurse, and it's usually one per customer."

Two days later, my assignment was to scrub alone for an appendectomy. Everything that could go wrong did. I couldn't remember the setup but, with The Voice yelling instructions in my ear, I managed semblance of order.

"Open the ties and first suture," my instructor bellowed.

I tore the end off a packet of suture, grasped the exposed needle and pulled. The suture unraveled its full length, and then escaping from the package, snapped back to its original shape. The momentum of this act, however, pulled the needle out of my grasp. The suture sailed across the room, hitting the circulating nurse on the shoulder. I tried a second time with the same results, although this time I hit the nurse on the forehead.

"At least his aim is improving," she muttered.

The towels and drapes slipped through my gloved hands like so much easy money (while pieces of suture wrapper adhered as if they had been grafted in place . . . I made the record for the number of knots in one length of suture). Finally, the patient was draped and the Mayo stand in position. The instruments on this tray were set in order of use. On the back left-hand corner was a small stainless steel bowl containing water. This was used to clean the dirty instruments when, and if, they were returned to you. I handed up the scalpel with a minimum of fumbling, retrieved and washed it. Then with wet, slippery fingers I tried to pick up a hemostat. This was like attempting to get a dime off a wet bar. I finally got a grip on it, only to have the instrument shoot out of my hand, fly across the room and hit the wall. The first instrument was followed by two more in rapid succession. The circulating nurse had become immune to flying objects and didn't bother ducking anymore. My instructor raised her eyes towards heaven and for once was speechless. The surgeon, who had obviously had student nurses inflicted on him before, said in a *crown of thorns* adjusting voice, "Nurse, if there is anything left on the tray that you think you can hold onto, please hand it to me." So, I handed him the bowl.

My next assignment was to observe an orthopaedic operation. I was enthralled by the tables covered with carpentry tools. Were they going to renovate the OR? As I hovered closer to the sterile tables, the scrub nurse became nervous.

"Do you know where the instrument room is?" she asked.

I did.

"Would you get me an Otis-Fensom elevator please."

I hurried to the instrument room. Here, behind glass doors was row after row of implements that would have made any medieval torturer feel at home. I searched for twenty minutes without luck, wondering why the name seemed familiar. Later, on my way to lunch, I stepped onto the elevator and suddenly realized the method that had been used to get rid of an overinquisitive and naive student.

The day came near the end of my OR experience when I was assigned to scrub alone for a bowel resection. The surgeon was notoriously fast. His assistant never arrived, however, leaving me with two jobs.

Between handing up the scalpel and the final dressing, a minor miracle took place. Every piece of information that had been drummed into my head fell into place. I anticipated the surgeon's wants. I also found I had a third hand when it was needed. After the patient was taken to the recovery room, I stood alone in the OR dismantling the setup.

"Well," The Voice said behind me, "How would you evaluate your performance for this operation?"

"I think I did O.K."

"You didn't do O.K." she roared, "You did an excellent job and you should be proud of yourself.

And do you know something, I was then and I still am.

Down the Tubes*

ETHEL GILLETTE, R.N., B.A.

As student nurses we were rich in textbook knowledge. We were adept at injecting oranges and could find any organ or muscle group on the lab dummies. We could follow the circulatory system like the River Nile on our charts. We wore the lips off Resusci-Annie with our CPR and those alcohol wipes, but hadn't yet been exposed to actual patients. And each day before our clinicals began, I would wonder if all this theoretical knowledge was going to make a difference in the *real* world. My eagerness to find out was mixed with fear.

The day finally arrived when we went to the hospital for our first clinical. I was lucky. My first patient was going to be discharged the next day and she seemed easy to care for. She had bathed earlier so I gave her a back rub with a soothing lotion. I made the bed so tightly, marked the place in her book where she was reading, brushed and combed her hair, and did her nails and tidied the room. The patient praised my care and it felt like wine—so heady. My first patient and she thought I was doing well. I couldn't wait until classroom time so I could boast. When I finished I washed her glasses, returned her book, and pointed to the spot she left off. I told her to just press her button if she needed me.

I went in a haze of pride to chart, but in about ten minutes her light went on. I bustled in and asked how I could help. She said, "I want my robe please." Happily I went to the closet to choose one of three she had hanging up. She said, "No, dear—I want the one I had on before my bath. It's my favorite because it's the

last gift my niece gave me. She was killed in an auto accident a year ago."

I stood frozen while she talked. Like a movie, a reel went off in my mind and I saw myself gathering up the sheets and the blue gown with them. I saw, like a horror movie, the linens and robe going down the laundry chute—down six floors to God knows where. The horror must have showed because the patient said, "What's the matter, dear?"

I said, "Would you excuse me a minute?" I went out of the room and saw my instructor coming down the hall and walked to meet her. She had told us to never leave the unit without permission from your instructor or charge nurse. I used to worry about being stricken with a heart attack and remaining on the unit, crawling, but *still there.*

I took a deep breath as I approached her and asked for permission to leave the unit. She asked what for. I took another breath and decided Truth has its place but this was *not* the place for it. I answered with this brilliant statement: "You told us to familiarize ourselves with the hospital. I have some time now, so I thought I'd start looking over the basement."

There was a long silence. I dared to look up from the floor and she said, "Gillette, what did you do?" That was enough to bring me to tears. I answered in a broken voice, "I just don't have time to stand here—my patient's best robe went down the laundry chute with the linens and I *have* to find it!"

* Reprinted with permission from Journal of Practical Nursing, ©1985; 35(2):37.

She sensed my despair and said, "All right—run—find the nearest stairway and run down to the basement. Don't waste time waiting for an elevator. Once the robe gets to the laundry the hot water and bleach will ruin it."

I ran. It was August in Florida and the stairway was not air conditioned. As a student I wore a grey cotton jumper, cotton blouse, white stockings, and oxfords. By the time I reached the basement, seven floors down, I was crumpled and damp. I walked through endless corridors and didn't see a laundry room. I met a young girl and asked her where the laundry room was. She said I would have to go to the maintenance engineer's office and tell him what floor and wing the linens were dropped from and he could then direct me to the chute opening. I went to his office, told the story and how I needed to find the robe quickly before the crew picked it up to wash.

He leaned back in his chair and laughed and laughed. After a very long time he finally stopped laughing and drew me a map. I found the door and when I yanked it open, laundry spilled out, piling high all around me. I was in a sea of soiled linen. By now I was in tears and told myself, okay, so what can they do to me if I can't find the robe? I'll buy her a new robe.

Then I remembered her words, "It's my favorite robe, a last present from my niece before she died in an auto crash."

With a determined sigh I began digging through laundry piles and pillow cases full of soiled laundry and emptied them, looking for the robe. By the time I opened the fifteenth pillow case I was thinking who wants to be a nurse anyway. I'll open just five more. After five more I said five more and that's it. It was suffocatingly hot down there; I was missing class and the robe was *not* in sight. As I opened the twenty-fifth sack, I said, okay five more and I mean it this time. The odor of soil, sweat and drainage was becoming overwhelming and they were not attached to persons so my gag reflex was beginning to work. (Later, as a nurse I learned that when you are caring for a *person*, concern seems to blot out odors.)

I spotted something bright blue in the bottom of the thirty-sixth pillow case. Feverishly I dumped the linens and there it was—the robe. I began stuffing things back and got the door closed. I ran up the seven flights. I reached my patient's room and went into her bathroom, washed the robe and hung it over the towel rack. I went back in, explained what happened and we both had a good laugh; hers from amusement, mine from relief.

Celebrity Musings*

LAURIE EYNON

If a chiropractor had examined Mozart,
would he have found a spinal chord?

If a geneticist examined Calvin Klein,
would he find designer genes?

If a plastic surgeon operated on Cheryl Tiegs,
could he fix her chic bones?

If an obstetrician examined Greta Garbo,
would he find a private womb?

If a dentist examined Sleeping Beauty,
would he find her cavity prone?

If a dentist examined Benji,
would he recommend a root kennel?

If an orthodontist examined F. Lee Bailey,
would he find he needed a retainer?

Physiology Exam†

CARRIE HENGESBACH

Where can you buy a cap for your knee?
Are there gems in the crown of your head?
Is the coat of your stomach tailor-made?
Will your shoulder blades cut bread?
If you wanted to shingle the roof of your mouth
Would you use all the nails of your toes?
Do you think that the arch of your foot is used
For a span of the bridge of your nose?
Would you say that your hands were a tropical land
Because some palms are there?

If you sailed the alimentary canal
Would you pass through the locks of your hair?
Do you think that the crook of your elbow
Will ever be sent to jail?
Or that the pupils of your eyes
At their exams will fail?
Could you build a ship on the slip of your tongue?
Who plays on the drums of your ears?
Who lives in the chamber of your heart?
Who discovered the fountain of tears?

Final Exams!*

SHIRLEY J. BRAVERMAN, R.N.

History   Describe the history of nursing from its origin to the present day, concentrating especially but not exclusively on its social, political, economic, religious, and philosophical impact on Europe, Asia, America, and Africa. Be brief, yet specific.

Surgery   You have been provided with a razor blade, a piece of gauze, and a bottle of Scotch. Remove your appendix. Do not suture until your work has been inspected. You have 15 minutes.

Psychology   2,500 riot-crazed aborigines are about to storm the classroom. Calm them using any coping mechanism you feel confident in using. Explain your reasoning.

Biology   Create life. Estimate the difference in subsequent human culture if this form of life had developed 500 million years earlier with special attention paid to its probable effect on the English parliamentary system. Prove your thesis.

Sociology   Estimate the sociological problems that might accompany the end of the world. Construct an experiment to test your theory.

Epistemology   Take a position for or against truth. Prove the validity of your position.

Philosophy   Sketch the development of human thought: estimate its significance. Compare it with the development of any other kind of thought.

Physics   Sketch the nature of matter. Include in your answer an evaluation of the impact of the development of the Band-Aid.

Political Science   There is a red telephone on your desk. Start World War III. Report at length on its socio-political effects, if any.

General Knowledge   Describe knowledge in detail. Be objective and specific. You have 15 minutes. (If you have any questions, raise your hand!)

How Not to Pass Your Exams*

KEN CORK

Do you suffer from exam nerves? Turn to jelly at the sight of an exam paper? Well, take comfort—there is always someone worse off than yourself. Ken Cork has been collecting particularly choice exam howlers over a number of years. Here we reprint a selection.

The skin provides an attractive covering for the humane animal and helps us keep our cool.

Transendential skin provides the bladder with three cells giving rise to watertight compartments at the base of which is a Trident.

Sebastian glands contained in the skin are often called pores, these pores are lined with erectile tissue which causes erection of the hare's follicles.

Straight cylindrical hairs are stronger than curly ones—on the other hand it can be that curly ones are flattened.

The skin can identify criminals, particularly if the detective is impressed with his finger prints.

The skin has collumns of cells arranged in the basement.

On the Care of the Eye and Blindness

The eyes of the patient are covered with a layer of skin which is only one cell thick.

The patient may be guided by lead dogs or the sticks that lead them.

If the retinue is transposed it can lead to a new site.

The person can fend for himself by the aid of a white stick which also acts as his sixth sense.

Books can be red if the person learns to write in Bailes.

The blind should be provided with radio and television sets.

In this age of terrorism, pullets entering the eye is not uncommon.

It must always be remembered that blind people are, in fact, human beings.

When the patient has learned Braile he can read the Dayly Papers.

The blind child will be able to see the advantages of attending a special school.

Some intense physio had taught him to see with his hands.

Gaynaecology and Obstrictive Practices

There are a lot of fairy tales related in the gaynae ward.

The gynae nurse may meet some queer conditions.

Gynaemen work closely with the obstrutitions.

The father or husband if any should be present to reinforce the insurance given by the nurse that everything is alright apart from loosing the baby.

Pauls tube, of course, has many uses apart from Colinsostomy.

Erotic gesticulation means that the woman had conceived.

Pre-operatively shave the gentle hairs and rape the part with sterile towels.

It is not surprizing that after exhausting labouring the baby's pulse is rapid.

*Reprinted from Nursing Times, ©1983; 79(51):58–60 with permission from Macmillan Magazines, Ltd.

Shells which are applied to the nipple so as to draw it out can be given to the mother when she has no milk.

The gynaecologist evicted a foreign body from the vagina.

The theatre superintendent said the patient was arresting and would need ventitilating.

The nurse must lend her sympathetic ear to the patients' problems including any sexual ones.

A full frontal X-ray showed some very interesting features of this patient's anatomy.

The Day the Nurse Discovered That

An auriscope was not what the stars foretold.

Aqueous humour did not mean laughing until you cry.

Hemicolectomy was not a form of punctuation resulting in a semicolon.

A pathologist is not a man who sits on one stool while examining another.

A uterine sound was not a baby crying for delivery.

Red corpuscles were not noncommissioned Russian officers.

Wet nursing was not exclusive to children.

Pan-hysterectomy was not an hysterical American air hostess.

A cystoscope was not an instrument with which one could get a closer look at the ward sister.

An HP was sauce that could talk.

A counterpane was not an analgesic.

Gynaecologists don't have male beds.

Photophobia was not camera shyness.

Ecchymoses was not just another swear word.

A Balkan beam was not a smile from a foreigner.

Ataxia is not an absence of taxis.

Some Notes on the Pill

This is an anti-fertility hormone and the morality of people taking it for purposes other than for which it is prescribed must be very questionable. It has, in fact, been blamed for much precautious conduct. Since its more liberal use the nurse must conceive the principle dangers of this contraception.

Little is really known about it but it can cause infertility but on stopping the pill the girl may become extremely fertile and produce many children all at once.

Patients on the pill can be said to be in a state of permanent pregnancy.

It is not unknown for it to produce a feeling of extreme insecurity in men whose wives take to the pill.

The nurse should always use a doctored prescription when ordering the pill.

Nursing School Days— Farewell*

CAROL WEIL, R.N.

'Twas the week before finals, and all through the class
The students were restless, and anxious to pass.
Home stockings are dirty; it's not we don't care,
But the laundry's not done yet because we're not there!
Our children are nestled in their unmade beds,
With dreams of home cooking and Mom in their heads.
And meanwhile, at Clinical, I, in my cap,
Had heard my assignment and wished I could nap.
When out in the hall we heard clapping and braying—
We thought our instructor was out there, role-playing!
Away to the doorway I flew with such haste,
I tripped on my notebook and fell on my face!
I was just sitting up and preparing to rise
When a crowd of nurse students appeared 'fore my eyes.
"Sit still; this will take 90 seconds," they said.
And proceeded to check from my toes to my head.
One straightened my airway; one looked for snakebite;
One shook me, and shouted, and said, "You all right?"
One tickled my feet, and one thumped on my chest.
One patted my hand and said, "Poor dear, just rest."
Then a gal so serene no mishap could affect her
(I knew right away 'twas the Nursing Director)
Appeared on the scene and said, "Hey, nurses! Move!
You've got patients to care for. Now get in the groove!
Now Penny! Now Ruthie! Now this isn't funny!
Your poor patient needs you; his nose is all runny.
That's care-plan material; write as you're rushin',
And have your notes ready for small group discussion.
There's lecture tomorrow; this clinic is done;
Now, dash away, dash away, into the sun!"

A kid meets me at home, saying, "Is your school done?"
I ask, "Who are you?" And he answers, "Your son!"
"How you've grown!" I exclaim, and my heart starts
    to flutter.
Then he asks, "What's for dinner?" I say, "Peanut
    butter.
I know you'd like roast beef, spaghetti, or ham,
But your Mom must prepare for the final exam!
Go look in the freezer; hey, just take a peek!
I'll fix that stuff soon, 'cause I'm done in *ONE WEEK!*"
That night, after studying, sleep came at last,
And I dreamed I was back at the school, in a class.
It seemed to be twilight; I looked left and right—
Then a woman appeared, from out of the night.
The Spirit of Florence! I drew my breath in,
Then I smiled, and I said, "Hi ya, Flo! How ya been?"
She spoke not a word, but went straight to her work.
She prepared me for finals, then called me a jerk!
"You think this was bad? And you're anxious to leave?"
Miss Nightingale said, as she laughed in her sleeve.
"Remember your school days; you'll not get them
    back.
Keep all those good memories safe and intact.
As time marches onward, and changes take place,
You'll wish for old friends, and for this rat race."
She picked up her lamp, and I picked up my book.
As we parted, I couldn't resist one last look.
I heard her exclaim at the top of her cords,
"Farewell to you all—and *GOOD LUCK ON YOUR
    BOARDS!*"

Graduation Day*

PAMELA F. RICHTER, R.N.

'Tis the day of graduation and all through my house
Shouts of joy can be heard from my child and
   my spouse.

For the past three years I've been getting an education
Always too busy, never took a vacation.

The dishes have been stacked in the sink with such
   care,
And no one in the house has clean clothes to wear.
That's because the dirty laundry is piled to the ceiling
Because I've been at school, learning about healing.
The dust bunnies have taken over my whole house
   as you see,
And the grass in the yard has now grown past my knee.

My daughter needed help with a report that was
   due soon,
But my report was due first, so I sent her back
   to her room.

And my family has been complaining about meals
   from the freezer,
So I opened some cans, but do you think that that
   pleased them?
They wanted to know why I never did cook,
And why did I always have my nose in a book?

Then my sister called to say she was in labor;
Asked me to come to the hospital because of
   the support that I gave her.
But I was working on a care plan that was two days
   past due,
So I asked her if she thought she could wait 'til I was
   through.

And my mother just called to say that I never
Come over to their house to see them, not ever!

Then my daughter wanted to know if we could go
   to the zoo,
But I said we couldn't because I had too much
   homework to do.

And my husband wants to know why we never
   go out,
And I said, "Right now, school work carries
   more clout."

Before each of my tests, I'd sit and study with Sue.
We'd eat lots of popcorn, and chocolate too!
We'd go through each chapter, and read all of our
   notes,
And then we'd go out for ice cream floats!

We'd study and study until we had it all down,
And I found myself wondering why I'd gained a few
   pounds.

And on a few occasions, when we were all
   tuckered out,
We wouldn't study at all, we'd just sit there and pout.
And then I'd go home to be with my family instead,
But by the time I'd gotten home, they had all gone
   to bed.

But now it's all over, graduation day is here!
And to my friends and my family who have all gathered
   here
I'd like to say now, "I'm finally through,
I couldn't have done it without you. I really love you!"

* Reprinted from Imprint, Vol. 37(2), April/May, 1990,
©National Student Nurses' Association, Inc.

The Board Game*

CONNIE MILNER, R.N.P.

I took the July Boards. Somehow, I didn't enjoy the experience. I was the first in my class to throw up. In order to spare others the slings and arrows, pitfalls and potholes awaiting them in the NCLEX minefield, what follows is a compilation of suggestions, observations and asides to help players get past the last of the first hurdles they must encounter as professionals to win the coveted state nursing license.

Don't fool yourself into thinking the test is easy because there are so many stupid people who have passed it.

Yes, you are expected to know everything.

To keep your friends on their toes, leave interesting facts or test questions on their answering machines.

Don't be surprised when you fail each practice test you take with uncanny consistency—count on a grade in the mid 60's—which will miraculously improve by test time. (This "BOARDerline" plateau is a mere stepping stone—accept it as such.)

Use the last of your student loan money to buy stock in Haagen Dazs, Steve's Ice Cream or Ben & Jerry's of Vermont.

Expect to make dumb mistakes in the face of sheer panic and terror.

Bring gum, candy, coffee, religious articles, lucky socks, fuzzy dice—whatever it takes to get you through this ordeal.

For the high spot of your two-day trial, make it a point to use the Porto-Sans at the test sites.

Because of the lengthy lines at these facilities, don't take Colace or Lasix the morning of the exam.

Once inside the portable john, don't look down.

Bring lunch and a thermos of anything—there seems to be a paucity of food concessions at test sites.

Arrive early (at least 30 minutes before showtime), just for the peace of mind.

Find as many of your friends as possible on the first morning of the test. Get on line together and you'll be able to sit within fainting distance of them.

Be aware that the test is numbered consecutively 1–372. Don't fall into the habit of thinking you're halfway finished at question 45 (that only works on Part I).

Wear a watch. Officials only warn you when there's 15 minutes left. By then, it's too late.

Know that Jesus, Buddha, Confucius, the Burning Bush and your Guardian Angel are there with you, but you're the one who has to take the test.

When filling in the appropriate answer circles, don't connect the dots or make happy faces inside the circles.

Learn "testspeak" regarding how to address patients and colleagues in the scenarios given (not to be confused with what actually is said on hospital floors under similar circumstances).

Don't let "BOARDom" set in or let your mind wander. Redouble your efforts to concentrate and see it through.

If you lose track of time, you'll know that you've reached the halfway mark when you hit the staples in the centerfold.

Don't listen to other people's answers after each test—you'll only get upset.

If you do compare notes with your friends, you'll find you got the bulk of the experimental questions right and the actual test questions wrong.

Don't anticipate euphoria at the end of the test. Expect fatigue, depression, anger and finally ambivalence.

If you're a pessimist, aim low and avoid disappointment.

Be aware that on the last test there wasn't one question on otitis media, Addison's or Cushing's diseases, or any of Freud's, Erikson's, Piaget's or Sullivan's stages.

Think of how better prepared you'll be for the next test in five months.

Be prepared to offer plenty to God in the bargaining stage of your post-test grief.

Try not to throw up on your "What Me Worry?" t-shirt.

Bring a mallet in case someone tells you it was pretty easy.

Find out when the LPN test is scheduled.

After the test, go home to relax. Unwind with a glass of wine—a "BOARDeaux" would be appropriate.

*Reprinted from Imprint, Vol. 38(2), April/May, 1991, ©National Student Nurses' Association, Inc. Edited from the original.

IT'S NOT AS EASY
AS IT LOOKS

Any new beginning is challenging and sometimes intimidating for most of us. Adjusting from the student role to the worker role is a humbling experience for many nurses.

A successful transition requires acknowledging that the norms and expectations in the academic world are very different from those in the clinical area. The new nurse will thrive in a climate that is conducive to learning and must become socially and politically comfortable in order to survive this new professional environment.

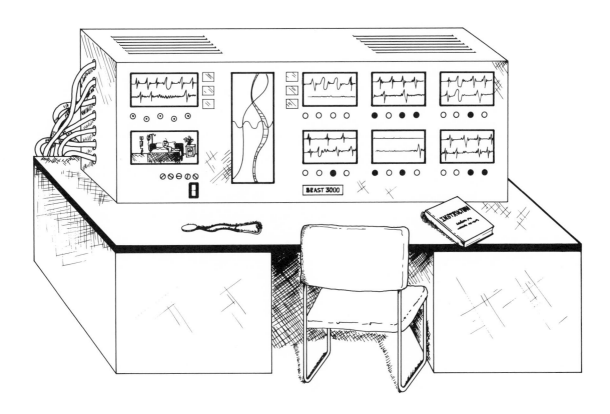

A Nurse's Guide to Recruitment Ads*

JILL CURRY, R.N., B.A., C.E.N.

I have stopped looking at recruitment ads. For one thing, I do not think I am their target audience. But the other day a "career directory" the size of a small city's telephone book arrived, and I could not resist the picture of an elderly, arthritis-riddled patient with the caption, "SHE NEEDS YOU," inspiring at the very least that long-overdue phone call to my mother and yet another setback in my resolution of codependency issues. Another ad read, "DO YOU CARE ABOUT NURSING?" I could apparently *prove* my commitment by responding.

Facilities always being expanded and showing off pictures of the flying buttresses, Ionic columns, or pseudo-Frank Lloyd Wright design of the facility must hope to fill their personnel offices with throngs of architecturally enthralled applicants. There was also a pervasive preoccupation with the "future." Recruits could expect a "great professional future." They would be on the "leading edge" of medical history. There is obviously an impressive payoff to come some distant day, but these ads made me a little leery for the here and now. I might be hit by a Mack truck on my way to work before the "future" dawns.

The prevalent theme of "diversity" often coincides with largess and inspired more anxiety than excitement in this potential recruit. As we balance our lives as spouses, parents, caretakers of elderly parents, and nurses, we have all the "diversity" we can handle, thank you.

Location. Location. Location. The descriptions would make the Chamber of Commerce proud. No matter where the facility is located, the ads sound basically the same:

"Located _____ (miles, states, light-years) north of _____ (major city, planet, civilization), _____ Hospital is nestled between the _____ (mountains, hills, plains, rolling countryside, toxic-waste dump) and the _____ (ocean, sea, lake, pond, factory outlet). The consistently mild climate, smog-free skies, and miles of beautiful _____ (beaches, nightclubs, traffic jams) make this a lovely area in which to live. Year-round outdoor recreation includes golf, tennis, and _____ (swimming, mass shootings, egg smelling); a rich and varied cultural environment includes resident professional theater, community orchestra, and _____ (town-fool competition, hog-calling, soap-carving exhibition). Educational opportunities such as _____ (MSN program, AMA-registered technician, truck driving) at _____ College or _____ University are enjoyed by all who live in our beautiful city."

Some of the photography rivals the Best of Show in any art gallery. Pictures of colorful hot-air balloons and rescue helicopters seem popular. I wonder if these may be the only way to get to work on time. Traditional images of nurses fluffing pillows are giving way to those of nurses leaning against, adjusting, or giving an inservice program on things like IV pumps. It is obvious that ad agencies think such high tech will attract nurses. All the scenes of happy nurses chatting in patient-less critical care units make me a little curious. Is the facility open for business? What is their mortality rate? Were they shut down by infection control? My personal favorite features a nurse looking sternly at the doctor and pointing to an open chart, as if to say, "You expect me to read *this* chicken scratch?!" Of course, the images of wide-eyed children gripping small stuffed animals have the power to stir maternal instincts in combat-hardened Marines. I would rather see a photograph of their in-house child care facility than these pictures of hospital administrators' children.

Much of the advertising for general hospitals strains the concept of truth in advertising. Nursing recruitment has spawned a new and complex language of persuasion. The *"Official Handbook to Nursing Opportunities," (OH-NO)* can help to decode words and phrases currently used in ads.

*Reprinted from Journal of Emergency Nursing, ©1991; 17(1):27A–28A with permission from Mosby Year Book.

Competitive salaries: Personnel managers of area hospitals put their heads together and fix salaries to keep each other competitive, hence the term.

Unlimited opportunities: "There are no problems, just opportunities." Be prepared for unlimited problems.

Teaching hospital: You will be responsible for making sure that the interns don't kill the patients.

Imaginative application of nursing knowledge: You mix your own IV fluids, mend patient gowns, and fashion hospital beds from trees you cut down in a nearby woods.

Flexible staffing: The flexible may refer to *you*. You might have to be adaptable enough to return to the hospital 20 minutes after working a double shift.

Career ladders: The rules regarding, and the paperwork required to achieve, any rung on this ladder exceed that required by the Internal Revenue Service for Donald Trump's tax return.

Sophisticated environment: There is germ-breeding carpet in patient rooms. Nurses are allowed to wear small earring posts on even-numbered Thursdays. This is also often a euphemism for big-city hospitals that don't give a hoot.

Collaborative working rapport between allied health professionals: Personnel from different departments no longer physically assault each other or call each other names in the halls.

We believe . . . nursing professionals should be afforded salaries and benefits they deserve . . .: We also believe that if wishes were horses, beggars would ride.

As a professional nurse . . .: *Un*professional nurses have different, more salacious, perks.

Progressive medicine: We will spring new and complicated procedures on you without warning, protocols, inservice training, or rationale.

Enrich your paraprofessional skills: Learn to identify hospital cafeteria food correctly at least 80% of the time.

Commitment to quality: We have no quality assurance department yet, so we will commit *you* to doing the studies.

Nurses take an interactive role in patient care: Feel free to ask another nurse to help you turn a patient.

Nurse-to-nurse network for clinical information and support: Our policy and procedure book is a little outdated, and our clinical educator is out on Workmen's Compensation for severe depression.

Our committee structure allows nurses to be a part of developing and implementing high-quality, patient-centered care: We expect you to come in on your day off for meetings.

A variety of nursing modalities are practiced: You have the choice of being assigned as the primary nurse for 30 patients, the team leader for 100, or the only nurse in the emergency department during a major disaster.

Providing an enviroment where newly acquired skills can be tested: For example, we will provide the opportunity to break the current record in the 100-yard dash to the blood bank, both with and without waxed floors.

Pay increases are based on a performance appraisal system: When you walk on water, you get a raise.

Promotional opportunities through dual-track ladder: That which goes up must come down.

We're proud of spending millions of dollars on improving our state-of-the-art facilities: We've put in a new wing of administrative offices; you can kiss goodbye any across-the-board raise within your lifetime.

Nursing practice is refined and perfected through input from management, education, marketing, and research and development: There are lots of people to tell you what to do; not one of them will be a nurse.

Voluntary hospital: We were originally a tanning salon, but we quite willingly converted to medical care where we could use much of the same equipment.

I have some suggestions of my *own* for those sophisticated Madison Avenue types. I would like to see:

"We will beat any other hospital's starting salary or city sanitation worker's wage by 10%."

"Free use of the rescue helicopter if your car is in the shop."

"Our night shift enjoys catered cuisine from Le Plume Cafe and the Imperial Chinese restaurant . . . and homemade desserts from the wives/husbands of top hospital officers."

"Each nurse has the privilege of annually targeting a physician of his or her choice for an IRS audit."

"Please excuse the lack of sophistication in our ad; we'd rather spend our money on nursing salaries."

Of course the best ad may be no ad at all. I would rather work for someone who has enough nurses already.

What the Ads Really Mean*

Despite the current uproar over job cuts, the number of nursing jobs advertised in *NT* each week is as large as ever. Here Mr. C. Handley, a Harrogate nursing officer, offers a tongue in cheek guide to what those ads *really* mean.

1. **"A small and friendly team."** This consists of a closely-knit group of nosey parkers, who will extend their friendship to you, wanted or not!

2. **"Required to undertake rotational day/night duties."** The important word here is "rotational." You'll be sent from days to nights to days. As long as your biorhythms are rotational you can apply.

3. **"Two minutes from the sea."** Obviously for the more marine minded. Non-swimmers should not apply.

4. **"To undertake duties throughout the hospital."** Today working in the operating theater—tomorrow, the boiler house.

5. **"This busy unit."** They would like others to join a group of willing individuals who are running round in circles, trying to get the work done.

How to Read the Job Ads†

Have you yet learnt to read between the lines of the job ads?

1. **"Recently up-graded theaters."** They got rid of the ether jar last week and repainted the doors.

2. **"A busy market town."** Do not work in the casualty department—market days can be hell.

3. **"Must have outstanding administrative ability and preferably some experience of catering."** The newly appointed district nursing officer will be expected to stand in when chef has one of his "off" days.

4. **"Typing ability an advantage."** Just why did the secretary leave? Ask the boss, or did he leave as well?

5. **"Two vacancies will occur."** Is there a coup planned?

6. **"Traditional nursing skills will never be out-dated?"** Quick, where did you put the leech bottles?

7. **"Situated in beautiful woodlands."** Beware! This place is in the middle of a dense forest, miles away from human habitation.

8. **"Vacancies exist for experienced pool nurses."** Those who only play pontoon, poker or backgammon need not apply.

9. **"If you wish to play a vital role in the developing field of . . . ."** You may work your fingers to the bone, but as soon as the first thing goes wrong, your head will be on the block.

10. **"A well-established hospital."** This hospital was built to cope with the expected wounded from the Crimea.

11. **"A maze of opportunities."** This really does describe the job opportunities for nurses well and is the one nearest the truth.

*Reprinted from Nursing Times, ©1983; 79(41):23 with permission from Macmillan Magazines, Ltd.
†Reprinted from Nursing Times, ©1983; 79(46):23 with permission from Macmillan Magazines, Ltd.

A Nurse Can Be a Man or a Woman*

ROSS P. MAYO

What was so terrifying in the nurse's station at Buchanan Elementary School? Me, a male nursing student.

It was during one of the rare occasions when Ms. Walker, the school nurse, momentarily stepped out of her office that I struck terror into one of the cutest little first-grade girls I've ever met.

Tammi skipped in with a tiny scratch on her finger. I looked up from figures of heights and weights I was recording and said in my usual businesslike voice, "Yes, how may I help you?" Apparently, to Tammi I sounded like the big bad wolf saying, "Come in, Little Red Riding Hood. I've been expecting you!" Her hesitancy to speak or come closer shocked me. No one had ever been afraid of me before. My uniform and supposed-to-be-there in the environment had stated plainly, "I am a nurse. I can help you. Trust me."

It took some time to convince Tammi that I was there to help, but she was not at ease until the familiar Ms. Walker returned and assured her that all was OK. Even then, she couldn't believe that I was a nurse. I asked her why. Her answer was simple enough, "You're not a lady."

I had encountered stereotyping and I decided to do something about it. I know I'm a nurse. My classmates and instructors know I'm a nurse. The other adults I come into contact with temporarily may be surprised, but eventually they realize I'm a nurse. I decided to make all the children at Buchanan aware that men can be nurses, that I was a nurse, and that men nurses are just as caring, competent, and professional as women nurses, whom all of us as children were programmed to expect in the nurse's office.

Time wouldn't permit me to speak to all the grades. I chose the second grades, because I believed seven-to-eight-year olds were the youngest age group fully able to understand what I had to say and why it needed to be said.

I asked the second-grade teachers to have their pupils write their ideas of what a nurse is. I then based a short talk on their answers. I thought the best way to involve the children was to make the task a "What's My Line?" type of game.

At the predetermined time, I arrived at a classroom in my disguise (an old flannel shirt and a colorful head band). I greeted the pupils and the teacher and asked their permission to speak.

I told the class I was there to talk to them after we played a game of "What's My Line?" I asked if there was anyone who knew me or who had seen me before. One little fellow named James raised his hand. I asked him to join me in the front of the class. As my assistant, he would have to tell his classmates when their guesses were incorrect.

I stated some personal background information, which would not reveal my identity. I mentioned that I rode motorcycles and raced my car at a race track with a sports car club. One boy shouted "You're a sports person. You're—Evel Knievel."

I gave my first clue. "Sometimes I ride in a special station wagon with the flashing red light on top."

James gleefully repeated, "No!" to guesses of policeman and fireman.

Then I gave the second clue. "I help keep people healthy." Nearly everyone jerked a hand high into the air. Everyone seemed so sure of his or her guess, but with James' first reponse of "no" to "doctor" all those sure expressions turned to confusion. After a moment someone guessed "dentist." With a big smile, James shook his head.

My next clue, "I help sick people get well," once again drew guesses of doctor. One little girl insisted that I was a doctor and that I was putting them all on.

When I stated I wasn't wearing my work shirt, someone then said, "ambulance driver." Before I could respond, I heard a faint voice say, "nurse?" Within seconds, the room was filled with giggles that turned into laughter.

Getting their attention once again, I said, "OK, my last clue is out in the hall and if it doesn't help, I'll tell you." While James went out to get Ms. Walker, who was holding my uniform top, I asked, "Why did you laugh when someone said nurse?" Amid another chorus of laughter I heard comments of "You're not a woman. You don't wear a white dress. You don't look like a nurse."

James returned with Ms. Walker and I removed my old flannel shirt and headband and then put on my uniform top. Someone still insisted I was a doctor. I asked, "Why do you think I'm a doctor?" Replies were, "You're a man. You have a doctor's shirt. Everyone knows that men are doctors." I then teased them once more by saying, "Someone already guessed correctly, but everybody laughed." What followed was a moment of silence and then a flood of astonished voices repeating, "A nurse! You're a nurse?" I told them that was correct and their not knowing was exactly why I was there to talk with them.

I pointed out how sex discrimination was apparently coming to an end in the professional occupations. I explained how both men and women are taking their places in nursing, medicine, law enforcement, and education. I explained what it means to be a professional, especially in nursing.

I related the story of terrified Tammi. I asked if they had any idea why she was so scared. One girl said, "My mom says never talk to strangers, especially men." To this I replied, "That's very true. It's also not a good idea to talk to strange ladies. But, who would be afraid to go up to a policeman you didn't know if you needed help?"

That question led me up to the point I wanted to make about approaching the nurse in school when necessary. I told them all they should get to know who the nurse was if they moved to another school.

Somebody then asked, "How can you tell a man nurse in the hospital from the doctors?" "More often than not," I replied, "a man nurse will be wearing a uniform like mine. He'll have a name tag on stating who he is and that he's a nurse. And if you ask a man nurse a question, he'll probably stop and answer you."

We then discussed how I got interested in nursing as an operating room technician with the Navy in Vietnam. This almost turned into the high point of the class, for young children usually enjoy colorful stories. I got the focus back to nursing in general by describing some of the many duties of a nurse. I related some of the things I had done. We talked about the various settings where a nurse might be employed and I added, "Some day I hope to be working as a nurse on a space station." To complete my presentation, I asked them to write down again their answers to the question, "What is a nurse?" A comparison of the before and after papers is enlightening.

Changes in Sex Stereotyping

Second-Graders' Views Before Class

"I think a nurse is a nice lady who helps people."

"A nurse is like a doctor. She helps a doctor. She gives us medicine. She works in a hospital."

"A nurse is helpful. She has white on her. She puts a Band-Aid on you when you are cut."

"A nurse is just like a doctor but she's a woman."

"A nurse may sit and watch a baby if a person is sick."

"Some nurses like to have a little bell and when the patients want the nurse she rings the bell and the nurse comes."

"If you are badly sick she takes you in the operating room."

Changes in Sex Stereotyping

Second-Graders' Views After Class

"A nurse can be a lady or a man. Nurses are working in clinics, schools, and hospitals. And some nurses are going to people's houses too. And a lady can be a doctor."

"She or he can work at home or factory or at a school. Always help you."

" A man and a lady are not the same. But there are some jobs that a man and a lady can do that are the same. And a nurse is one of them."

"Nurses don't just work with doctors. They work by themselves."

"They help doctors sometimes. They help people on their own. They work in a hospital or in the Navy. They work almost anywhere."

"They won't scare you."

"Nurses baby-sit babies when mothers are in the hospital because men are horrible cooks."

"When you go to the hospital and see a man nurse do not be scared. They help you."

Of Caps and Shoes*

DELAILAH KHAN, R.N., B.Sc.N.

During my years of studenthood I managed, through a combination of fate and luck, to evade situations in which the wearing of a nursing cap was required. Many of the clinical areas assigned to me were not conducive to the donning of such headgear. For instance, it would have been difficult to maintain an air of proficiency with a cap propped under an O.R. hood. And, in contrast to days gone by, our lecture outfits were jeans, sweat shirts and bare heads, rather than full uniform.

My nursing cap was kept well protected by stretchy plastic wrap on a bookcase shelf. There it sat as a symbol of my profession. It was the recipient of many admiring comments from those who came to borrow books. However, it was not something that I had any intention of wearing. I would not need it to identify myself as a nurse. After all, I had white shoes.

This aversion to headgear, of any type, even followed me to my graduation ceremony. I had visions of my mortar board careening onto the lap of some dignitary, after a sure-to-happen trip (literally) across the stage. Luckily, when the time came, some degree of decorum was maintained—I tripped bareheaded.

Time passed. The world beyond studenthood became the real world and suddenly I was an R.N.—a Real Nurse. My greatest fear, which until this time had been treated with calculated denial and avoidance, would soon be realized.

"Our nurses wear full uniforms here," the supervisor said.

I felt the color ebb from my face. "Er . . . that includes a cap?" I stammered. Somehow I knew she wasn't just referring to both parts of a pant suit.

"Of course," snapped the supervisor, "full uniform!" At this point she was probably thinking of hiring someone with better hearing than mine.

My dreams of taking the nursing profession by storm and forever changing its course were shattered. Before my first shift nightmares ran like open I.V.'s.

Scenes of my frazzled cap dangling in yards of traction or falling with tremendous flurry into a sterile field hovered in my subconscious. Onlookers invading my dreams bore only contempt. Their caps stayed in place as if permanent fixtures! Upon awakening, I desperately searched for signs of sickness. I prayed for dysentery, but all was in vain.

With prayers unanswered, I pondered my dilemma. I felt adept at balancing a full bedpan; I could fill a syringe without contamination; and I never got urinals mixed up with icejugs. Technically, I was not awkward. But as I stared at my cap, *sans* plastic cement, all confidence vanished. Two hairpins stood between me and a career in paint-by-numbers.

Seemingly without warning, the moment arrived. It was time. Like a tightrope walker balancing a fruit basket on her head, I maneuvered my way to the nurses' station. All eyes were on me (of course, the fact that the other nurses were simply wondering who I was did not matter. It was the cap!)

I had just spent 15 minutes locked in the bathroom agonizing with comb, pins and cap. The comb bared its teeth at me as I attempted to subdue strands of unruly hair. My troop of sweaty hairpins and my unpatriotic cap did not make the battle any easier. Suturing was a definite possibility, but since my threshold for pain was almost non-existent, I decided against it. In those few minutes, hours passed. Finally, I was able to affix the cap to my head—how long it would remain there was questionable. At least it was the night shift; the lights would be dim.

I had lost the battle, but I put away the thoughts of this personal problem to get on with the matters at hand. Adrenalin that had been coursing through my system while I struggled in the bathroom was put to use. The floor was busy and, in between getting acquainted with the area, staff and patients, I dealt with the usual havoc of the night shift.

* Reproduced with permission from The Canadian Nurse/L'infirmiere canadienne, ©1984; 80(8):46.

As morning approached, I was passing out (not me, but my medications) when one of the patients commented on my appearance.

"You look very unruffled after such a busy night . . . very professional," he said.

I returned his smile and knowingly looked down at my white shoes. To my dismay, I discovered that the bedpan I had dropped earlier had not quite missed my shoes!

"Yes," he said, looking somewhere above my head, "those caps look great!"

My fears had not come true: no snaking traction had snared my cap and gravity had curbed its appetite for propelling it groundwards. I had overcome this worry, and like most fears, it seemed quite laughable . . . after the fact.

Now, about those white shoes . . .

Transparent Benefits*

JILL L. CURRY, R.N., B.S.N., C.E.N.

"No, please, don't take it away," I screamed. The two men looked at me in surprise.

"Where are you taking it?" I asked, tears in my eyes.

"I think they are going to ship it to some hospital in South America," said George, as he placed it in a cardboard box filled with popcorn-shaped packing material.

"Can't you let it stay here just a little longer?" I begged. "The new one is not working out at all well, and I've heard we might go back to the old one."

"Sorry," George said. "We have our orders. I'm afraid the new computer system is here to stay."

He gave me a comforting pat on my shoulder. Then he picked up the box with my old friend in it and left.

I had semi-hidden the old terminal beneath a little-used desk, hoping somehow it might be called back into service. I could not accept its inevitable retirement.

I had mastered the old computer in less than 15 minutes when it was introduced ten years ago. Now, after three months of figuring out the vagaries of the new, improved computer, I longed for the easy simplicity of the old "blue box" which had served so well. Sure, the old computer had its faults, but it understood me. It would gladly present a menu of options when I typed in an ambiguous request for a chest x-ray. With the push of a button, I could select portable, single or multiple views. And I could count on the speedy delivery of the order to the appropriate department.

Now all orders are given code names World War II military intelligence personnel would have been proud to claim, such as CXRROUT (routine chest x-ray). The new system does not allow for mistakes. Leave out one R and the system simply denies such a test exists and threatens to disable your user number. The old "blue box" would never have treated me so badly.

The introduction of the new computer system sorely taxed everyone's patience and diplomacy. It nearly turned the emergency department, if not the entire hospital, into a long-term care facility. Lab tests that used to be back within 30 minutes took two hours to complete.

Without warning, a mysterious link in the computer system, known as the INTERFACE, would slow the transmission of orders to the lab. Of course, this would happen during the busiest times in the ED. By the time the slowdown was discovered, the diagnosis, treatment and disposition of patients would be hopelessly delayed. Orders apparently lingered in an area of the universe best described in certain religious circles as limbo, rendering ED and laboratory staff at each other's throats.

Sometimes an order simply disappeared, or would be translated into a different order. A new computer

* Reprinted from Point of View, ©1990; 27(1):16–17 with permission from Ethicon, Inc.

term began being bandied about by the experts in data processing, hereafter referred to as DP. The term PHANTOM became the official name given to the culprit responsible for these occurrences. It was at this point that I strongly urged the employment of a priest to exorcise the ills of the system, or at least a consultation with the neighboring community of mediums and psychics. My appeals fell on deaf ears, and we struggled on.

Urine cultures seemed to be most vulnerable to arbitrary termination by the computer. Patients would call for culture reports, only to find that the computer had canceled the order without notice. Ten incident reports later, the personnel from DP acceded to the fact that this was a significant enough problem for them to address. A week later, a solution was proposed. Another new term was introduced. We were promised that if urine cultures were ordered EXPEDITE instead of the familiar STAT, ROUTINE or PRE-OP, we could expect the order to be processed. We tried this for a week.

Another five incident reports later, DP conceded that this was not enough. Now they suggested that every laboratory test, including urine cultures, be ordered as LAB COLLECTIBLE. Since when did laboratory personnel ever coax and collect urine specimens from patients? But we swallowed our pride and faithfully noted *yes* when the computer asked this question.

Another three incident reports later, DP realized that urine cultures were still being thrown out by the computer. The newest dictum demanded that we put a urine sample in a culture tube for every urinalysis sent, whether or not a culture was ordered. This worked well until we ran out of culture tubes. Central supply had to submit a rush order to the company who makes the tubes, greatly increasing the company's revenue, but not our own.

It bothered me that the ordering of lab tests now required at least three times more discrete tasks than with the old system. Additional numbers and data were necessary in the manual labeling of all specimens. (The computer is not capable of generating preprinted labels.) Once I facetiously added the maiden name of a patient's mother to the label on a urine specimen, but no one noticed, much less appreciated, the desperate attempt at humor.

I realized during the all-too-brief training session that the new computer would require considerably more nurturing and care than the old machine. I asked, with blasphemous assertiveness, how the new system was to benefit caregivers, specifically nursing personnel? Indignantly the trainer stated there were "transparent benefits," and left me to ponder this obscurity. I later decided the "transparent benefits" and the PHANTOM were somehow related.

The plastic cover added to the computer keyboard reminded me of the cash register at the local sandwich shop. Could it be that DP was afraid the computer would catch some germ or, worse yet, some computer virus from us? The implications were downright insulting.

DP said nothing could be done about eliminating the infamous "caps lock" button. This button served no purpose except, when accidently pressed, to banish the current user with a sign flashing ILLEGAL ENTRY. East Germany should have such security. Why it was placed so close to frequently used keys, deliberately inviting trespass, could only be explained by the condescending and sadistic glee with which DP came to rescue us.

Three months later, we reached a détente with the new computer that Henry Kissinger would admire. We are now getting laboratory results back in a timely manner, sometimes faster than we did with old "blue box." We have the capability of retrieving the results of tests done several days earlier, something we could not do with the old system.

The PHANTOM seems to be at bay, like the Loch Ness monster returning to the depths of the lake. And we have resumed our usual good relations with the laboratory people.

I no longer hiss at the computer terminal each time I pass it. I can order most common diagnostic studies without referring to the cumbersome and nonindexed computer manual. I can even replenish the printer paper, and I have mastered changing the ribbon. I can undo the mistakes of less computer-skilled personnel. And I speak with DP personnel in a more civil tone. But I still keep an eye on the travel fares to South America.

E.D. Gazette*

SUSAN MOORE, R.N., B.S.N., C.C.R.N., C.E.N.

Once Upon a Busy Day at Triage

"Hi. Can we help you?"

"I sure hope so."

"What can we do for you?"

"Make me better."

"What's the matter?"

"I don't know. That's why I came to you."

"What brings you to the hospital today?"

"A cab."

"What symptoms are you having?"

"Symptoms?"

"Are you feeling badly?"

"Of course. If I felt good, I wouldn't be here."

"Do you have pain?"

"Well, not exactly."

"What are you feeling?"

"Blah."

"Please describe it."

"I can't exactly."

"Are you sick to your stomach?"

"Well, I was . . ."

"How long has this been going on?"

"Oh, goodness. My Aunt Grizelda came to visit in the summer of 1967. I think that was the first time this happened. Or was it in 1976?"

"And you've had this feeling ever since?"

"Oh, no, nurse. That's a pretty dumb question."

"It comes and goes?"

"Yes."

"How long has this episode lasted?"

"Well, this time it hasn't been as bad—up until this morning, when it got worse."

"What have you done for it before?"

"Sat it out."

"How come you came in this time?"

"I'm tired of it."

"Have you taken any medicine for it?"

"No."

"Are you allergic to any medicines?"

"Yes. Oh, does aspirin count?"

"You're allergic to aspirin?"

"No, I took a few today."

"How many?"

"Oh, not more than 10 or 12. Codeine."

"You took codeine, too?"

"Toxic Sock" Syndrome

A nursing survey made its way through the department a while ago. One question was easy to answer: "What do you like least about emergency nursing?" "*Feet*," I said. "Foul feet, to be specific; toenails are extra."

I regularly amaze peers with my ability to remove every stitch of clothing and leave shoes in place. Total body assessment, contrary to what you have been told, does not include the area below the ankles. The posterior tibial artery is palpable above the shoe line.

I've suggested a moat to the emergency department. It would be shallow, would be filled with warm, sudsy water, and would completely encircle the unit. The administration has scoffed at the plan, but *they* don't have to deal with feet (a few heels, maybe.)

Please, no offense to the persons with less-than-rosebud piggies. As my kids and pets can well attest, I can claim no perfumed digits myself. My nursing shoes are left outside on my arrival at home; the cat *loves* them. I always drive home with the utmost caution. Heaven forbid that I'd arrive unconscious and awaken as some overzealous nurse is removing my shoes. "Oh no!" I'd gasp, as he/she fell back with a grimace. The world would know that the nurse with the foot phobia is a victim of "toxic sock" syndrome herself.

An Ode to Scrubs

Actually, I've always had a hard time getting to work clean, even before I reproduced. Some folks are innately tidier than others; they probably have a mutant gene somewhere. Unfortunately, neither of my children had

* Reprinted from Journal of Emergency Nursing, ©1986; 12(1):18A–20A with permission from Mosby Year Book. Edited from the original.

a chance to receive this gene; their father certainly does not possess it. My DNA goes without saying.

Nursing is full of challenges. Getting two kids to a day-care center and my body to work, unstained, is just one of them. I usually fail, but I weather my failures in a sophisticated manner: I pretend I haven't noticed the Ovaltine cascade down my scapula: "Stain? Well, I'll be darned! Wonder how that got there."

If the stain can't truly be ignored, I attempt the "rinse it in the sink while still wearing it" maneuver. This leads to large wet spots in embarrassing places, with a drying time of 2 to 4 hours.

Now, any stain obtained in the line of duty is another matter. Blood stains not entirely rinsed are somehow noble; at least you haven't been charting *all* day.

My life has been revolutionized by the arrival of scrub suits in the department. I'm blessed by the fact that my body was designed for "scrubs." Or they were designed for my body. Years ago, the future scrub-unit manufacturers of America must have toured the hospital, searching for the typical nurse body. There I was. "That is the typical nurse," they said, "narrow on top, wide at the bottom. Let us design scrubs to cover that bottom." Behold, scrubs were born.

Heard in the Emergency Department

"Next of kin? George Brown. I believe he's the administrator here."

"Did you notice any of those little crawly bugs when you pulled off my clothes? They've been driving me crazy lately."

"Oh, not more than 15 or 20 aspirin since last night."

"You know, the last time they tried to start an IV, the doctor ended up doing a little operation here in my elbow."

"I'm allergic to everything but Dilaudid."

"You're only a nurse?"

"I called an ambulance because I didn't have any money for a cab. You have to admit me because I don't have a way home."

"I feel safe with an old nurse like you around."

"I'll bet I'm the only patient you know who has successfully sued a nurse for malpractice."

"Why don't you go get that pretty nurse over there to come take care of me?"

A Study in Vein

Dear Patient: I understand that sometimes you don't get very straight answers when you want to know how sick you really are. If that is the case, please follow Sue's simple formula for health status determination. Count the number of tubes attached to your body. The number is directly related to the severity of your problem. As a rule, more than one tube and you're sure to be admitted; four or more, and you're destined for intensive care. (Note that each lumen on your pulmonary artery line counts as one tube.)

One can be even more technical here. Count the number of pieces of tape on your IV site. The more tape, the lousier your veins. The number of sticks it took to endow you with that tube is not always a reliable indicator; every nurse has to learn sometime, and even experienced nurses have a bad day now and then. No matter how many pieces of tape you have, be brave, dear patient, and accept your fate. We can't all be 19-year-old construction workers with garden hoses on our arms.

Over the years, I've made a study of veins in America. This is the only significant correlation I can find: overall, the harder it is to start the IV, the more the patient needs it.

A patient-vein classification system has been difficult to create, but after much arduous concentration, I present the following:

1. Veins belonging to the man of my dreams (described at the end of the second paragraph).

2. "Pudding wrapped in tissue paper" veins: little blue lines that burst at the slightest nick, leaving gigantic hematomas that never go away.

3. Veins of young teenagers so healthy that they don't need veins and consequently have none.

4. Dreaded "turtle reflex" veins belonging to remarkable individuals who can retract their veins in fear, more or less involuntarily.

It Still Makes
Me Cringe*

NEAL BUCKLEY, S.R.N., R.M.N.

If I were to ask the question: "Have you ever done anything at work that made you wish the ground would open up and swallow you?," I think most nurses would admit to something.

I asked my colleagues if they could recall their own embarrassing moments and found myself bombarded with tales. So, for nurses everywhere, here are a few of the best stories.

One nursing auxiliary, who had been in the job but a short time, created a splendid floral effect for a patient's locker—in a glass urine bottle.

Putting things into the wrong orifice seems a popular theme with beginners—for instance, the aminophylline suppository inserted in the nostril, or the Senokot tablet given rectally.

Then there is the pre-operative shave. How many nurses will own up to having performed a full pubic shave on a patient about to have surgery on an in-growing toenail?

One nurse recalled her first time in a busy surgical ward. On being asked by Sister to shave a patient in readiness for theater, she produced what she thought was a perfect result. Her pride was soon shattered, however, when she was shown the note sent by the surgeon. It read: "Will the nurse who shaved this patient kindly note that I like to make my own incisions."

A staff nurse explained how, on his first day in a new ward as a student, he was asked to escort a patient to the x-ray department. Having secured the patient safely aboard the ambulance, he proceeded to run a quarter of a mile to meet him at journey's end. It was only when the ambulanceman asked him why he had not traveled with them that he realized what a fool he had made of himself.

Patients with parts of their anatomy missing often provoke embarrassing incidents, such as the occasion when an enrolled nurse was asked to get a patient dressed and into an armchair. She searched high and low for a missing slipper, then discovered that this particular patient had only one leg.

I can remember, as a student, going fully equipped to the bedside to cut a chap's toenails and, on pulling back the bedclothes, found—yes, you've guessed it—he had no legs.

Hospital equipment sometimes develops a mind of its own that leads to some interesting situations. I heard a tale of an electro-cardiograph machine that could not be switched off until a full roll of paper had been discharged over the bed, and a bath lift plus patient that got stuck three feet in the air. And then there is the one about the sphygmomanometer cuff that inflated like a Christmas balloon and popped.

Thermometers, in particular, have been the bane of many a nurse's existence. Take, for instance, the nursing auxiliary who, on being asked to clean the ward thermometers, promptly doused 30 of them in hot soapy water and broke every one of them.

One student nurse recounted the time she decided to clean the false teeth of an entire psychogeriatric ward. She scrubbed them vigorously until they shone like polished ivory. But giving them back to their respective owners proved difficult—she found she had scrubbed off the patients' names.

While waiting for the tutor, a nurse on her first day in introductory training happened to notice an elderly disheveled-looking man wandering around in a confused manner. She approached the man with an offer to provide a helping hand back to the geriatric ward.

"No, you may not," came the indignant reply, "I'm the senior tutor!"

One unsuspecting charge nurse telephoned a relative to let him know that his father had been transferred—

* Reprinted from Nursing Times, ©1990; 86(50):27 with permission from Macmillan Magazines, Ltd.

as previously discussed—to a home for the elderly. His choice of words could have been better, for when he said: "Your father has gone . . . ," the person on the other end of the line burst into tears and exclaimed: "He seemed fine last night."

Finally, a Sister, while showing a group of learners round her ward, was asked if any of the patients were ever violent towards staff. "Never," she replied. Then within a few seconds, she was being battered about the head by a manic elderly lady.

How to Survive a Building Project*

ELLEN GORE, R.N., B.S.N.

Probably most hospital employees have endured at least one building project. How did you survive? Let's examine the steps of survival for those employees whose hospital is about to embark upon an expansion, remodeling or a completely new building.

There is one prerequisite: You will be asked to donate towards the new building. Keep your checkbook or payroll deduction slip handy as this is standard operating procedure. "This is your hospital so we want you, the employees, to have a part in its construction." This is a favorite line. A little, a lot, whatever you can spare for the next five years is appropriate. Besides, it does make a good tax deduction, so be prepared to give until it hurts. Later on, in a couple of months, you can change your mind and cancel the payroll deduction, but you will have been a part of the "giving society." Maybe you will believe in the project and continue your donation for the designated time. The decision is yours.

Once the initial monies are obtained, be on your guard. Strange noises, yawning pits and monster machines will one day appear in your life with no warning. You will not be issued a hard hat. But you should consider your own purchase of earphones, earplugs, a ghetto blaster . . . anything that will drown out the noise. Don't worry about the patients: you can't hear their requests anyway. They soon learn to take care of themselves, write messages, or leave as soon as possible.

For a while, watching the workers dig holes is fun as they dig such nice big ones. Then, you begin to realize that giant holes surround the hospital. What are they planning, you wonder? Is this an invasion by the construction world? Will the entire building disappear into the holes? Are they building a moat? The next thing you notice is that all the windows are being boarded up with wood. Why? Then, you figure it out. They are building a floating box with real surprises inside . . . people!

Remember that entrance to the hospital you have used for the past five years? Well, find another one as that entrance is history. A machine needed a parking space, so the entrance was torn down. You can't find another entrance? Just keep walking . . . there must be one. (Or you can be airlifted in via a skylight.) Look for others wandering around with dazed looks on their faces and join them. Sooner or later someone will realize that you are hospital employees looking for a way in to work, and will help you find a narrow cave-like passage into the building. Of course you may be arrested for loitering, but at least you will be off the streets.

Once you get inside the building you know your way around, but don't forget those poor unfortunates . . . the visitors. They may wander for days if no one stops and gives them directions. "You can't get there from here anymore," strikes terror in the heart of a husband trying to get his wife to the labor and delivery suite in time.

*Reprinted from Point of View, ©1988; 25(3):18–20 with permission from Ethicon, Inc. Edited from the original.

Jackhammer serenade will be your theme song. You will eat to the beat, feel the earth move beneath your feet, and maybe even have to dodge a falling ceiling as the jackhammers keep working around you. Look up, down, around and behind you before moving. Otherwise, you may suddenly be surrounded by men with hammers removing the ground upon which you stand. To be fair, the men using the jackhammers do not have it easy either. They are used to the noise and cannot understand why an operating room supervisor calls their boss all excited because the noise is over a room in which eye surgery is being done and the entire room is vibrating. But they do cease as requested. However, they begin again the next morning. The request to cease is relayed once again and they comply. Why can't construction work be done after surgery hours, say from midnight to four in the morning? We work shift work . . . why not them?

The emergency department will begin to have a rash of seasonal disease . . . rubberneck syndrome. Giant cranes will be moved into position and hospital staff will be busy looking up watching the monsters doing their thing. When the show is over the rubberneck syndrome will begin. Not only will sore necks be a problem, but so will those sprains, breaks and bruises caused by looking up and not watching where one is walking. Holes in the ground will trap a lot of unsuspecting rubberneckers. A good rule is to watch where you are walking and to stand still if you are going to look up. Otherwise, you may be finding out just how good your hospital's emergency department really is . . . first hand.

A lot of fun can be had during construction. Remember, the work being done has to have workers. They are usually young, good-looking and love ladies. In their macho world, women are to be whistled at, teased and maybe even asked for dates. This can be a two-way trip, ladies. We women also can whistle, tease and ask the opposite sex out. It is fun to watch the workers' reactions when the tables are turned. Besides, anyone in their right mind enjoys being thought attractive, regardless of which sex they are. It is so much nicer to go to work thinking you are gorgeous instead of reliving a fight with your spouse or children.

Unusual Occurrences

Unusual happenings can occur while you are on duty during the period of construction. Let's look at a few incidents.

You are busily caring for a patient. Just after you and the patient have moved away from the bed, the entire ceiling over the bed comes crashing down. After both of you stop shaking, you get on the phone to the construction foreman.

You rudely tell him what has happened and what you think of the entire building program. By the time he gets to where you are, you have calmed down and can show him what has happened. He is as upset as you are. Everyone is frightened for what might have been. Suppose the patient had been in the bed . . . a skull fracture or worse would have resulted. How did the accident happen? Seems the construction occurring around the patient rooms involved movement of heavy support beams. One was dropped and fell through the ceiling. So that is the pipe sticking down! Feeling ten years older and a lot grayer, you explain the problem to the patient and cross your fingers that something similar will not happen again. So does the foreman. The patient requests another room in another wing.

The operating room staff has some fun moments too. While busily changing and chatting in the women's dressing room one afternoon, hearing male voices causes the women to look skyward. They have an audience looking down upon their clothes-changing. Duct work you know. Everyone is a little embarrassed, but this show is over. However, on another day, the ceiling is out in the bathroom and a few more compromising situations occur. The operating room's female staff is now a little leery of even going into the change room. The construction workers are taking bets on what their next scenes will be. The construction foreman has apologized and promised it won't happen again. But his credibility is sinking.

You and your friends decide to go to lunch in the cafeteria. You meander down the usual corridors and suddenly discover a solid wall where the cafeteria used to be. Voices can be heard through the wall. Is there another entrance? Are there signs directing you? What are the voices saying? Maybe you are freaking out? After standing around complaining, your group decides to ask for assistance and begins looking for someone to ask. You are the only people around. You retrace your steps. Eventually you find an administrative person to ask. He snarls about a memo that went out two weeks ago changing the entrance. "Must be having a bad day," you think as you go back to your starting point, find and read the memo, then start out again. Success . . . the cafeteria is found. You get your lunch, find a place to sit, and then glance at the clock . . . horrors! You have five minutes to eat and return to your unit, so you cram and run. About one hour from now your lunch will land with a thud and you will need antacid help. Stress management anyone?

Nursing service calls and asks you to stop by for a discussion of your duty hours. You arrive at the usual location, but no offices are left . . . just bare walls. Again, there were memos alerting the staff to the move, but who reads all those memos? You decide you had better start, or you won't be able to pick up your paycheck as the payroll office may move too. Where will it end?

Finally your work is done for the day. You head out the nearest exit for the parking lot. Upon arrival at your brand new vehicle . . . guess what? It is no longer in a parking space, but it is sitting up on what used to be a lawn with a gigantic dent in the side. There are no notes on the windshield. You begin to fume. Storming back into the hospital, you find the person coordinating the building project and unload your venom. He lets you finish. Then he says, "We wondered whose car it was and figured the owner would come yelling when the dent was noticed." You stand there trying to say

something, but you are so furious all that comes out of your mouth is a stammer. You then learn you must see the construction foreman, as a giant crane backed into your car. Seems there were supposed to be "No Parking" signs in that area, but they were never posted. So, who pays for the damage to the car? If you are lucky, you may have an answer in a couple of months. For now, you have two options: one, you can patiently await the settlement, or two, you can nag the hospital and the construction company until they finally do something. Whichever option you choose, it will be stressful for you. Nagging can be more fun; however, patience may win you more kind thoughts. You will probably still have to wait the same amount of time, so take your pick of the options.

Grand Opening

For five years you have endured thinking the end will never come. But suddenly, one spring day, the machines begin to leave. Parking spaces appear miraculously. You see announcements about hospital grand openings. Can the construction really be finished? Yes. You have survived!

The Olympic Athletes of Mill Town Memorial*

ANNETTE RHODES, R.N., B.S.

With all the excitement in the air during this Olympic year, I could not help but reflect on some of the outstanding athletic feats I have witnessed being performed by members of our own staff here at little Mill Town Memorial. I am moved to accord them the honor and recognition they deserve:

First place in Pole-Vaulting should definitely be awarded to Ivy Tubing of Central Service, who, using a nearby mop handle, neatly vaulted over the lower half of Central's French doors in pursuit of an orderly making off with an unrequisitioned enema bag.

The gold medal for overall accomplishment in Track and Field should be awarded to Moe Mentum, Medical Imaging Transport Technician. Moe recently laid 24 feet of wheelchair tracks on the wet wax in the back hallway before he was overtaken by several irate members of the housekeeping crew. He was subsequently decorated for his achievement in the field behind the hospital.

The Nursing Staff of 3E Orthopedics definitely deserves the gold in the Discus event, having managed (last month alone) thirty-two patients with slipped, herniated, and/or ruptured discuses, while keeping their own discuses in proper alignment. Honorable mention in this event is merited by Tab U. Late of Data Processing, though his discuses were just a tad too floppy to take first place.

Outstanding in the Shot Put competition was ICU Nurse Posey Beltt, who deftly sank 29 intramuscular injections in a single shift—all of them in the old gluteus maximus bull's-eye!

Lab Staff are unsurpassed at the Javelin Throw. Lab assistant Turna Kett recently managed a venous draw on patient Billy Rubin without even entering his room. How's that for blood and body fluid precautions?

Neurosurgeon Crane E. Otomy, on the other hand, is extremely proud of his excellence in the Long Jump. Just last Tuesday, the good doctor cleared the steam tables and the salad bar from a standing start in the kitchen. It must be added, however, that much of Dr. O's inspiration for this amazing feat arose from the sharp end of dietary supervisor Lotta Hash's roasting fork. (Lotta is easily peeved by kitchen intruders.)

ER Physician Dr. Cox Oydde recently broke his own record for the 50-Meter-Sprint, when he dashed from the ER to a 03:00 Code Blue in ICU. Cox faced possible disqualification, however, when it was observed that he had forgotten his scrub pants in the rush. Concern was that this might have lent him unfair advantage in terms of wind resistance. Since the Code was a success, the complaint was withdrawn. The crowd of spectators roared their approval of that decision—and of Cox's performance!

Top honors for the Hammer Throw are due Jerry Riggs of our Engineering Department. Jerry accidentally whacked his thumb while tacking up a "Don't Litter" sign in the front parking lot, slinging his hammer a record breaking 250 feet, and taking out the windshield of the brand-new BMW of orthopedic surgeon, Dr. Cal Caneus. Dr. Caneus' plans for returning the hammer have not yet been announced.

The nursing office supervisors would make prime competitors in the 100-Yard-Dash. Supervisor Addir Pose rapidly responded to 37 pages in one recent PM shift alone; while runner-up Minnie Mumwork came in second with 31.

Polly R. Thritis is definitely our Decathlon champion. On January 14th, Polly single-handedly removed 12 Foley catheters before her morning coffee break! (She also should win an award for getting a coffee break!)

The Accounting Department would knock our socks off on the Balance Beam. Accounting clerks Adam Upp and Cal Q. Late can juggle those budget figures better than any one around!

Another area in which we truly shine is the Horizontal Bar exercises. Community feedback indicates

*Reprinted with permission from Journal of Nursing Jocularity, ©1992; 2(3):24–25.

IT'S NOT AS EASY AS IT LOOKS

that several of our staff members have been found horizontal in any number of local bars and drinking establishments. Only discretion keeps me from mentioning their names. Good show!

Grabbing the gold in the 3000-Meter Steeplechase was our own Dee Posit, credit office clerk. Dee cleared her desk and three swivel chairs in her pursuit of patient, Adam Steeple, who—upon discharge—refused to pay the bill for his bunionectomy.

Highest honors for the Broad Jump are unanimously awarded to a male member of our staff who prefers that I not mention his name. Descriptions of his athletic achievements are detailed on the wall in the men's locker room.

M. T. Shelves and his all-girl Boxing team from Purchasing can take the gold, silver and bronze in that event. The medals, unfortunately, are all back-ordered.

And lastly, we all feel that Director of Nursing, Meg A. Fone, is unsurpassed in qualifying as the world's best in the Trap Shoot, having more experience in shooting off her trap than anyone we know.

Twenty-Two Laws They Wouldn't Dare Enforce*

ROBERT W. PELTON

Nurses prohibited from dipping snuff while on duty? From shaving a man's chest? From taking a nap in a refrigerator? From shouting at a patient to awaken him in the morning?

Samuel Johnson once said: "The law is the last result of human wisdom acting upon human experience for the benefit of the public." See if you can fully agree with this bit of philosophy after considering these examples of strange legislation tailored specifically to govern nurses' activities, both private and professional. Then decide for yourself!

Let's look first at laws about nurses' looks. The town of Carrizozo, New Mexico, strictly forbids a nurse ever to appear in public unshaven. This particular old law applies to her legs as well as her face!

Speaking of legs, an ordinance in Bristol, Tennessee, prohibits nurses from stopping in a hospital hallway to straighten or pull up their stockings. A similar law in Denison, Texas, spells out the penalty to be imposed for adjusting stockings in any public area of the hospital. To violate this law, to commit this "lurid act," can get you up to 12 months in jail. (I wonder whether pantyhose will require a separate law?)

Nurses' appearance apparently troubled lawmakers in Morristown, Pennsylvania, too. There, nurses are required to buy a special permit to wear any cosmetics. It's against the law to put on make-up without written permission. The fine when caught: $15.00. And in Oklahoma, no nurse is allowed to do her own hair. She must, according to this old law, be licensed to do her hair by the state or face prosecution. (Do you suppose an Oklahoma nurse could be thrown in jail for wearing a wig without a license?)

A city in one of Oklahoma's neighboring states— Missouri—also has an oddball law on its books. In Calloway, an ordinance prohibits a fireman from rescuing either nurses or their patients from a fire in a hospital unless they are fully dressed. No nurse attired in a nightgown may be assisted, nor may any patient in bed clothes. Clothing is also the object of a law still on the books in Fosterdale, Wyoming. The old ordinance bans a nurse from walking down any hospital hallway while wearing body-hugging dresses. A $25.00 fine can be imposed on any nurse who wears "clothing that clings to her body."

And in Wyoming's neighbor—Utah—policemen in the town of Glover will check out another part of your attire: your shoes. An ordinance in Glover limits the heel length of an on-duty nurse's shoes to one and one-half inches.

Shoes also dominated the thoughts of lawmakers in Cleveland. There, nurses are prohibited from wearing patent leather shoes while on duty. The law sternly warns that men "might look at the reflection" in the shoes and thereby see something they shouldn't.

If that law is geared to safeguard nurses' morals, consider these two: In Nottingham, South Dakota, nurses cannot initiate a conversation with a married man under 20 years of age. And the pithy wording of an ordinance on the books in Buckland, Alaska, declares, "Any person shall not tempt any married nurse."

Personal habits come under legal scrutiny elsewhere. How about the old snuff-dipping law in Winchester, Mississippi? Nurses are outlawed from using snuff while on duty at a hospital. And they can't smoke pipes or cigars either. But in New Pine, Arizona, it's against the law for a patient to give a nurse a cigarette. Male patients can't even offer a nurse a cigarette, nor can they smoke in her presence.

If you happen to be thirsty and in Cornwall, Wyoming, don't expect to be able to walk up to any bar and

*Published in RN April 1976, Vol. 39(4), pages 39–41. Copyright

---

IT'S NOT AS EASY AS IT LOOKS

order a drink. Nurses in Cornwall are banned from drinking within five feet of a bar in any public place. And try to stay away from Corvallis, Oregon, if you happen to be a coffee-drinker. There is a strict curfew: Nurses are expressly forbidden to have a cup of coffee after 6 P.M.

Other strange laws address themselves to what must be regarded as nurses' professional activities. For example, it is a felony in Brogan, Montana, for a nurse to open and read a doctor's mail. She isn't allowed to read mail even if she has been given permission to do so by the doctor! South of there, in Tryden, Colorado, nurses are not allowed to shout at a patient to wake him from a sound sleep. To do so brings a stiff fine! And in nearby Arizona, nurses in the little town of Saturno are prohibited from shaving a patient's chest. Nurses who do are subject to a fine.

Three other laws truly deserve to be classified as "unique" in their own right. In quiet little Banrose, Louisiana, a local ordinance states that no nurse—whether on duty or off duty—may sleep in a refrigerator. Nurses in Warburg, Minnesota, are prohibited from hanging their freshly washed lingerie on a clothesline in the hospital. And the community of Hoppersville, North Carolina, prohibits nurses from wrestling in the hallways of the hospital. You are not allowed to wrestle no matter how angry you might be. (Presumably, however, you may punch, pull hair, scratch, bite, bend, fold, or spindle without running afoul of the law.)

Finally, here's one strange piece of legislation that just might appeal to you: In Carson Springs, Tennessee, a local law bans all patients from sticking their tongues out at nurses. Even making faces at any nurse on duty is specifically prohibited too.

These are but a few of the odd situations covered by strange nursing-oriented statutes and ordinances that I've found around our country. Most of these laws were passed and then forgotten many years ago—as a matter of fact, city officials in some of the cities cited expressed astonishment when I told them that the laws existed in their communities. Some statutes have been repealed by collective or blanket legislation. But others are still on the books and, hopefully, forgotten in today's jet-age.

Henry Ward Beecher says it all when he sums up his view on the joyful art of lawmaking: "We bury men when they are dead, but we try to embalm the dead body of laws, keeping the corpse in sight long after the vitality has gone. It usually takes a hundred years to make a law; and then, after the law has done its work, it usually takes a hundred years to get rid of it."

ANATOMY AND DIAGNOSIS

As on any other work day, nurse Linea Joint drove her new Lamina Lateralis from her home in Musculi Beach to Saint Basalis. After change of shift, she realized that this day would be trachea than most.

Her patient, Margo Frontalis, fell off a trapezium and was brought to X-ray. The technician loaded the filum into the camerae, et septa the focus was Broca. She tela Dr. Ramus Dexter that there was no rima reason the machine was caput.

After work, Linea went to dinner with Crista for a tunica sandwich and a large pepsin. To relaxin they decided to go to the Saint Vitus' Dance and meet the old ganglia.

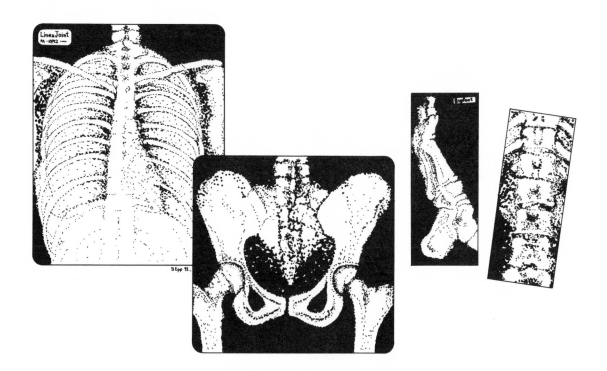

Medical Terminology for the Layman*

Artery—The study of paintings
Barium—What you do when CPR fails
Caesarean Section—A district in Rome
Colic—A sheep dog
Coma—A punctuation mark
Congenital—Friendly
Dilate—To live longer
Fester—Quicker
G.I. Series—Baseball games between teams of soldiers
Grippe—A suit case
Hangnail—A coat hook
Medical Staff—A doctor's cane
Morbid—A higher offer
Nitrate—Lower than the day rate
Node—Was aware of
Organic—Musical
Outpatient—A person who has fainted
Post-operative—A letter carrier
Protein—In favor of young people
Secretion—Hiding anything
Serology—Study of English Knighthood
Tablet—A small table
Tumor—An extra pair
Urine—Opposite of you're out
Varicose veins—Veins which are very close together

A Cilia Tale There Is Yet to Tell†

JENNY ASHMORE
PAUL GARDNER
KAREN WALKER

We went to St. Pancreas Station to catch the Eustachian Tube to Marrowbone. As we left, another train was renin alongside.

My traveling companion was Polly Peptide, who is a gland woman.

I had a bile of banknotes in my pocket to buy our tickets to the Islets of Langerhans.

On arrival at Marrowbone Station we saw one of Epi's taxis, so Polly said that we had better iris car.

We bought our tickets at the travel agents.

As we left, Polly decided that she wanted to go to Westminster Abbey to hear the organ of Corti.

However, I dropped my suitcases in the road where a car ran over them and rectum. The driver got out and grabbed hold of Polly, so I told him to liver alone. After much persuasion, he left.

By now we were well and truly lost, so I asked a passer-by to draw us a diaphragm. He told us to enter the Buccal cavity and turn left by the Pillars of Fauces.

*Reprinted from Plastic Surgical Nursing, ©1988; 8(1):29 with permission from Anthony J. Janetti, Inc. Edited from the original.
†Reprinted from Nursing Times, ©1979; 75(13):555 with permission from Macmillan Magazines, Ltd.

But we had no more chyme; the pain was due to leave.

We dashed to the airport, where Polly peptin to the "ladies" to powder her nose.

"Where is she?" I asked rather sternum, and as she appeared eyelashed out with a verbal attack.

On the plane, we met some interesting people; one man was a jugular who was rather vein about his occupation. His son was also in the circus, and spent most of his time on the trapezius.

Another man, who was rather boring really, thought his own jokes rather humerus.

The pilot, Carpine, had rather constricting views on flying. His stewardess, Angie O'Tensin, was rather vagus about her job.

The engines (made by Occulomotors Unltd.) were turning over, while the pilot took time to testes instruments. Once ovaries problems, we took off.

We came across another circus act on the plane—a couple called the Duo Denum.

One little boy brought his tortoise collis.

There were some animals in the hold, and the ganglions could be heard roaring ferociously. Polly put some cotton wool in her ears Psoas to block out the noise.

An announcement came over the tannoy: "Will Master Cates please come to the galley."

"Ear I am," I said as I approached Angie.

"Oh good," she said, "Perhaps you would take the coffee round for me."

After I had put on my pinna, I went back into the gangway, bearing my wares.

Suddenly, a man slipped off his seat and lay prostate on the floor.

A punkrocker was on board called Sid Viscerous, with his PR manager. They both laughed at the man's predicament.

In fact, the man went hysterical, so Angie told him to pull himself together, stand up and make a clean breast of it.

As he was explaining, Polly arrived on the scene, quite worried as to my whereabouts.

"Oh urea, I was getting quite concerned about you."

"My dear, urine quite a state, go and sit down again, I won't be long." I said—I didn't know she cared!

Just then, the electrolytes went out. Because it was dark, Billy Rubin sprained his ankle; he slipped on a carotid under a seat. We told him not to lose his temporal as he lymphed back to his place.

A glint caught my eye. It was the reflection from the well styloid bracelet Polly was wearing. I knew where she was then, so I put down the tray and went to her side.

Over the intercom, we heard the pilot say, "I sphincter's something wrong."

To keep up morale, Sig. Moidcolon did his act, which resulted in many smiling faeces.

Polly said she felt ileum—she was often squamous during air travel.

The flight continued, uneventfully. The hydrochloric power was restored and all was peaceful.

That was until we passed over the Calyces and ran into a carpal tunnel. However, the turbinates gradually decreased as we descended through the clouds.

Polly shouted to me, "Isn't that Little's Area in the distance?" She was right.

It was not long before we prepared to land.

A taxi took us to our destination, the Pia Mater Hotel, which was situated on the beta side of town.

Although the traffic was noisy, we could not hear much from our rooms which were well insulined.

Our holiday was a dream come true. Long days were spent on the breach absorbing vitamin D.

On the chewsday, we took a bone arrows and played artery.

That evening, in the Lum Bar, we were listening to the hotel's headwaitress Emma raging at the barman, when in walked the singer Peri Stalsis, who was on holiday with his guitarist Cy Napse. They agreed to meatus for dinner and talus about their experiences.

The day we left, we had one last dipin one of the hotel's many pons.

We will never forget our trypsin that week, and decided that we muscle again.

"See If They Are A Live"*

KAREN M. JORDAN, C.O.R.T.

Working in surgery, I often see patients who have received inappropriate emergency treatment prior to hospitalization. Unfortunately, this may increase the pain and the extent of the injury and decrease the chance for a favorable outcome. In an attempt, albeit small, to combat this problem, I teach emergency care to Boy Scouts working on their First Aid Merit Badges.

I simplify the material I was taught in an Emergency Medical Technician course and combine this with the required reading in the Scout publications. However, despite my best efforts, the answers the boys give on their tests sometimes bear little resemblance to the material I presented. Often, the spelling is incorrect but sometimes, the problem lies much deeper.

While I stress direct pressure as the treatment for severe bleeding, they've answered that if pressure doesn't work, apply a "tarniquit," "tiniquit," "tinyquot," or a "tourniquot."

When someone has been bitten by a dog, you should "make sure the dog doesn't have rabies, if he does go to the doctor, if not just clean him with soap." Or "a. get the name, b. get the doctor, c. get the dog." Another boy suggested "a. get the dog. b. get the info on the dog tags to see if it has rabies," and "c. bring it and the victim to a hospital."

The boys often go camping and must be prepared for emergencies they might encounter in the wilderness. I asked them what they would do if they got a fishhook stuck in their finger. One boy answered "wait till the doctor gets there." This seemed impractical until I remembered that his father is a pediatrician.

They practiced splinting fractures or dislocations and on the test they were questioned about the "rule" for splinting. I was advised "don't forse the bone and always splint stiff."

They also practiced ways to move someone with a back or neck injury. When asked about it they said to "take three guys and put them at feet, wast, and head then pull them up slowly and keep him straight." However, the definitive answer must be to move him "carefully, slowly, and if possible dont."

If a person is choking "do the squze," "the stomach squeeze," "Himlik hug," or "himlick huge."

Upon encountering an unconscious person "check to see whats rong and if brething." They said to "check for breating and hart working."

Cuts and injuries that are not life-threatening can be treated in many different ways. Either "clean it and put stealie pad on," "Put a goz pad on," or "press a wet cloth on it and yell for help."

Snake bites presented quite a challenge to my fledgling first aiders. One said to "cut out the bite area and slow down the victoms blood." He didn't explain how to slow it down—one can only imagine the possibilities. Another said to "cut a y shape in the biteen place and suck the vimon out." You can also "tie some string above the bite or suck the vimen out only if you see it." If string doesn't work this first-aider might—"use a suction cup to suck out the poison and make little slits in the skin, tie a rope above the bite."

Even with all of this valuable medical advice, before you can follow any of it you must check and "see if they are a live."

* Reprinted from Today's OR Nurse, ©1984; 6(8):36 with permission from Slack, Inc.

Anatomically Speaking*

ETHEL GILLETTE, R.N., B.A.

Licensed Practical Nurses . . . Has your axis been spinning? Have you had a pain in the cervical? Have you felt a decided slump in your lumbar and thoracic? Have the horizons of your coccyx and sacrum been widening lately? Have you found yourself leaning heavily on your ocranan? Has your malleus, stapes and incus been invaded by thousands and thousands of words? Have your ciliary muscles been overworked; with your rods and cones busy, busy? Does your mandible hang open a lot? Has the epidermis of your frontal been deeply furrowed? Do you feel like crowning just anybody's coronal lately?

Well, just hang onto your lambadoidal and close your mandible; hang onto your axons; don't dent your dendrites and never snap your Synapse. You just have the summer blahs. August is here and the air is hot and heavy. The year seems long and unending. Summer storms erupt suddenly, savagely and many times without warning. Just as the storms pass, summer will end suddenly. When it is gone you will mourn it and wish you had enjoyed it more.

So it is with your summer blahs and your perception of your role as a L.P.N. Close your mandible (mouth) because the fact that you're reading this article proves you're using your cerebrum. It means you are a professional. A professional needs to keep informed. What better way than the combined benefits of membership in your National L.P.N. organization and access to a monthly journal—a journal that not only informs you of what is happening in your profession, but *also* provides factual, informative articles. Remember strategy, planned strategy is far superior to just spinning our axis.

The saying "Alone we fall, united we stand" has a message for all L.P.N.'s. Leaning on your ocranons may support your bodies. It certainly does not lend itself to support of our profession or L.P.N. organization. Slim down your coccyx and sacrum and widen the horizons of your profession with active participation. Belong to your National Federation of L.P.N.'s because it *is* a small world. What happens in New York, Alabama or Wyoming can affect L.P.N.'s in states far away. Be active in your local organization. Keep it a quality organization with your valuable input.

Summer will soon end and fall will follow. As L.P.N.'s the summer blahs I mentioned earlier will end, only to be followed by problems, decisions and choices that may make summer problems nostalgic losses. Isn't that great, challenges, challenges! As L.P.N.'s you never seem to lack them. Perhaps that is why L.P.N.'s rank high in flexibility. As your skills increase naturally, pressures and decisions also increase. It would seem logical that you would get increasing pains in the cervical (neck). Two aspirins and going to bed will not take away that pain. Head on confrontation of problems followed by thinking them through is one step. Next, a discussion at your local L.P.N. monthly meeting will give you a chance to get valuable input from other L.P.N.'s.

Summer blahs will soon be over but challenges and problems are forever. So, just hang on to your lambadoidal and close your mandible; hang on to your axons; don't dent your dendrites and never snap your Synapse because challenge can and should bring out the best in you.

*Reprinted with permission from Journal of Nursing Care, ©1980; 13(8):7.

Why Do I Always Misdiagnose the Patient I Know Best?*

SANDE JONES, R.N., M.S.

There's a well-known medical saying: "In diagnosis, think of the easy first." But many nurses I know think of the most difficult—or the most dreadful—first. I myself am a prime example.

Let me assure you that I'm not new to the world of nursing or medical diagnoses. Over the past 14 years, I've worked as a primary nurse, team leader, float nurse, relief nurse, assistant head nurse, and instructor. I've dealt with cardiac arrest, pulmonary edema, eviscerations, and patients in DTs. I've even learned to use more than 50 formal nursing diagnoses to describe my clinical findings.

My nursing experience plus the baccalaureate and master's degrees I earned along the way taught me all there is to know about clinical diagnosis. I couldn't possibly miss the obvious—or so I used to think.

The first clue that I might not know it all came when I realized I hadn't had my menstrual period for a while. "Has it been one, two, or three months?" I wondered. "Never mind," I reassured myself. "It's probably because I've been careless about taking my birth control pills."

Thus I diagnosed my problem—*Non-compliance with the medical regimen*—and went on about my business. To be sure, I started to get a little nervous when people asked me about the weight I was gaining, but I simply attributed this to *Altered nutrition, more than body requirements.*

Just to make sure I wasn't pregnant—*Health maintenance alteration*—I bought one of those pregnancy test kits. When the results were interpreted as "not positive," I decided that I must have an ovarian tumor.

After reviewing my textbooks, I made an appointment with a gynecologist. I told him exactly how I thought he should deal with the tumor. I even told him when I wanted to be admitted for an exploratory laparotomy.

He kept giving me blank looks. Then he handed me his stethoscope and asked if I'd like to hear my baby's heartbeat. I was stunned when he said I'd deliver in five months.

I finally agreed with his medical diagnosis, and used sarcasm to avoid the nursing diagnosis: *Coping, ineffective individual.* When people asked if I was pregnant, I said, "No, I swallowed the med cart."

As days whizzed by, I continued my work, took Lamaze classes with my husband, and gathered all the books on baby care that I knew I'd get around to reading before the baby arrived.

Then one Saturday morning, while talking to a neighbor, I felt a trickle running down my legs. "Good grief," I thought, "Now I have incontinence or *Altered patterns of urinary elimination.*" As the day progressed, my incontinence increased and I developed a terrible backache—*Altered comfort: Pain.*

By evening I was in the bathroom every 10 minutes, and the back pain was worse. I pulled out my nursing textbooks, carried them to the bathroom, sat on the toilet, and tried to figure out what was wrong. As soon as I saw the words, "renal calculi," I thought, "That's it. I'm passing a kidney stone."

I called the hospital and asked to speak to the emergency department's physician on call. He listened patiently as I poured out my signs, symptoms, diagnosis, and possible treatment. I heard a sigh just before he asked, "Are you a nurse?"

Naturally, the physician urged me to come to the hospital immediately. The 26-mile trip seemed to take forever. My husband, remembering our Lamaze instructions, asked, "Don't you think you should start working on some of your breathing techniques?"

"No," I yelled. "I'm having a kidney stone, not a baby."

The emergency room staff took one look at me, put me in a wheelchair, and whisked me away to the maternity floor. I kept telling them I needed an IVP, but they insisted I needed L & D.

When I finally allowed an OB nurse to examine me, she said, "You're going to deliver very soon."

"You must be mistaken," I told her. "I can't have the baby today. I'm not due for another four weeks. I have classes scheduled for the next three weeks. I'm going to shop for diapers and a crib next week. And I promised the anesthesiologist I'd deliver on a weekday so he'd be here to give me epidural anesthesia."

By the time I finished explaining to the hospital staff why I couldn't possibly be having my baby that day, my obstetrician had arrived. "You're all ready to go," he said.

"No, I'm not," I replied defiantly. "I will not go into the delivery room until I know I can have epidural anesthesia to prevent labor pains."

He assured me that the baby would arrive before the anesthesiologist, and that I shouldn't worry about labor because it was almost over.

It was. My next surprise was when the doctor showed me a darling little girl with a mop of black hair. I knew she couldn't be mine because all the indications were that I was to have a baby boy with blond hair. He finally persuaded me there couldn't be a mistake because I was the only one to deliver that morning.

The Brotherhood of Motherhood*

SUSAN MOORE, R.N., B.S.N., C.C.R.N., C.E.N.

"Oh, it's very simple to cure diaper rash," I'd blithely say, "just let the little one run around the house without a diaper." Was I crazy? What did I think diapers were *for*?

How my advice to parents has changed. The metamorphosis began, I believe, about 5 years ago, around the time I brought my first child home.

"What?" I used to say, a faint note of disdain in my voice, "You gave your child Tylenol *before* you checked his temperature?" (I'd nearly "tsk tsk" out loud). "You mean you gave him the amoxicillin you had left over from his last ear infection? Well, that's why it came back, you know" (sigh). Now, I do know. If you get the tid dose down 5 days in a row, you have accomplished a miracle. Normal moms then dwindle down to bid, then qd, then qod, then the bottle sits in the fridge until the child has a fever again. Then—pop, pop, two Tylenols and a good dose of amoxicillin to last him until morning. That's real life.

I remember telling mothers, "Your baby just has a little gastroenteritis. Her system needs a rest. Just give her clear liquids for the next 24 hours." HAH! Sounds fine in theory. But what if that baby gets better in 8 hours? No amount of Pedialyte is going to make the little darling happy. Mom will surely have given in to something solid by morning.

I used to know very well that you let a child with a fever run around in as little clothing as possible. But parents always looked at me as if I had lost my mind when I suggested that they not put the sweater, coat, hat, scarf, and blanket on the little tyke to take him home. *Now* I know why. There is a hormone, possibly a genetically programmed instinct, that forces parents to swaddle their children. I *know* better and it *still* takes all the willpower that I can muster not to put just one more thin fuzzy blanket on the little guy at night. I now feel that I've achieved a great victory if I can convince parents to use sleepers without feet in them.

Oh, the disdain I used to feel when parents would bring in little Sally at 3 AM, obviously still covered with yesterday's dirt. ("Don't they at least *bathe* the child before bedtime?") Well, if I had a dollar for every time *my* children have gone to bed dirty, I could afford a nanny to bathe them *for* me.

I remember the times I would carefully secure a Band-Aid to an 18-month-old's arm, cautioning the parent to leave it there for 24 hours . . . Hah again! That Band-Aid was off before the child hit the parking lot. Now, put a Band-Aid on a 4-year-old and the problem comes when you need to pull it *off* a week later to remove the sutures.

And how *could* that mother of a 2-year-old be so negligent as to allow her child to drink gasoline? She probably blinked or paused to tie her shoe—that cruel, uncaring woman! Oh, and now I know that there is no such thing as a child-proof cap (adult-proof, yes); these are only challenges to be overcome.

I remember very clearly Sister Flanahan, my instructor, saying in her most nursely tone, "The diligent nurse should always suspect child abuse when the parent's story does not fit the injury." Of course, the story NEVER fits the injury. My kids have had falls that should have broken every bone in their bodies; they didn't even pause to cry. They also have bruises that no one, not even their little selves, can provide a history for. The universal laws of cause and effect do not apply to children. Noooo, you have to rely on other evidence. In fact, the more bizarre the story, the more likely it happened, just that way.

I suppose after all, that motherhood has done me some good. I'm kinder to other parents for it and, possibly, a better nurse. I'm also frequently late for work, have peanut butter on my pants, and sing "Hokey Pokey" under my breath until my colleagues could scream. It's experience that no nursing textbook could ever provide.

*Reprinted from Journal of Emergency Nursing, ©1988; 14(2):123 with permission from Mosby Year Book, Inc.

Diagnosing the Cat*

LINDA M. NORLANDER, R.N., B.S.N.

I am a nurse—registered and licensed. I carry my own malpractice insurance. I know what words like thermomandibular and myocardial infarction mean. I know where the islets of Langerhans are. My children are very impressed.

My husband is an upholsterer who also knows where the islets of Langerhans are. He's not that impressed.

From time to time the children come to me and ask, "Mom, since you're a nurse, what about such and such?" I try to dazzle them.

"The frog died of massive cerebral trauma, contusions, and abrasions." (The frog was squished under the lawnmower.)

"Dad has a headache because of sinus congestion and allergic rhinitis." (He's sneezing his head off because it's hayfever season.)

"Your brother is in bed because of a febrile condition brought on by an influenzalike virus." (He caught something that was going around.)

In the past year I have successfully diagnosed an appendicitis attack and a broken elbow. (I admit I missed two strep throats and one ear infection. My husband figured those out. I prefer flashy diagnoses, anyway.)

One day the children asked, "What's wrong with the dog?" (Most of what's wrong with the dog is that he's dumb.)

"The dog has minimal brain function because of arrested development in the fetal-to-infant stage."

"No really, Mom. Why is he doing that?" The dog was dragging his hindquarters across the carpet with a determined look.

"Children, the dog is suffering from the pain and itch of hemorrhoidal tissue."

Weighing my options (which included taking him to the veterinarian) I decided to give him a sitz bath. I took the dog to the basement and sat him in a tub of warm water, thinking all the while of new mothers who also have sore bottoms. The dog never forgave me, but my standing with the children rose.

Then, the next spring, a new case challenged me.

"Mom, what's wrong with the cat? It looks like it swallowed the basketball."

So I put on my nurse's cap and went out to examine the cat, who was a vagrant trespassing on our deck. It did indeed look as if it had swallowed the basketball. A quick look ruled that out: the basketball was under the deck. So I made my diagnosis and gathered the children around me.

"Children," I said solemnly, "I think the cat is very sick. Its stomach is big from built-up fluid due to renal failure. Kitty will probably just go out into the woods and die." I told them a transplant was out of the question. I told myself this was a lesson in how nature takes its course.

The cat's stomach got bigger and bigger. Then, sadly, the cat did go out into the woods. But the next day the cat came back—with six little renal failures in various shades of black and grey. My credibility, like the President's, had been damaged. How was I to know the cat was a female?

The cat went into renal failure one more time. The children didn't ask me what was wrong with her this time. After that, we took her to a registered, licensed veterinarian for some serious family planning.

I no longer practice veterinary medicine without a license. In fact, like the President, I'm trying to keep a low profile. If the children have a question, I send them to my husband. He has no problem saying, "The dog is doing that because he's dumb. The frog is dead because it got run over. Your mother has a headache because she thinks too hard. . . ."

Bon Voyage?*

ANDREA KOVALESKY, R.N., M.S.N.

I'll never figure out how the airlines guarantee that Nurse Ann, as my family calls me, is always booked on the flight where someone gets sick.

I have examined my tickets carefully for some code that identifies me as an RN—to no avail. I have even considered, as a last resort, demanding health certificates from my fellow passengers before boarding. Don't get me wrong—I'm proud of my profession and I'm eager to help anyone in need. But being 36,000 feet in the air with only an oxygen tank and a glass of water at hand is just not my idea of the ideal health care setting.

My first in-flight emergency came during a brief interstate flight. As I was resting comfortably, my job in the hospital far from my thoughts, a stewardess came up the aisle quietly asking if anyone on board had medical training.

Suddenly beginning to feel ill myself, I announced, "_____."

"What?" she asked.

"I'm a nurse."

"I still can't hear you."

"I'M A NURSE!"

"This way, please."

The patient was a middle-aged man breathing with great difficulty. He was traveling alone. Another stewardess had already started giving him oxygen, but he still seemed restless and in distress. Somehow I remembered how to take his pulse.

When, between gasps, the man informed me that he was on his way to the university for a heart transplant, ischemia set in—in me. I sat with one hand on the patient's wrist, the other holding my watch in front of me, and my eyes fixed on his chest, thinking, "Don't arrest. Oh God, please don't let him arrest." Despite a pulse of 156 for the patient and a close 124 for me, we both survived the landing. The waiting ambulance whisked the man away.

I approached my next few flights with caution, but they were uneventful. Then it happened again. The stewardess asked me to keep an eye on the man across the aisle who was acting a bit strangely.

"Oh no," I thought. "This is it. He's got a gun and he's getting ready to hijack the plane." So I started a vigil of intense observation and imagination.

Gradually, I realized that my "suspect" was not a hijacker but someone experiencing a psychotic episode. I relayed my assessment to the crew. During the movie the man stood up and could not be made to sit down.

This time, however, I was not alone. There was a physician on board, although one who, in the midst of our efforts, confessed his uneasiness: "You see," he said, "I work in research."

"Wonderful," I replied. "I work in the nursery."

Nevertheless, by pooling what little psychiatric training we had, we managed to settle the man down.

I have one other complaint regarding flight nursing. Not only are the working conditions less than ideal and not only does my anxiety level increase fourfold—but I never get a follow-up report. Whatever happened to those people who had to put up with my glazed eyes and trembling hands? I'll never know if the first patient survived his transplant operation or if the second arrived alert enough to greet the familiar faces waiting for him.

But I *do* know that I like nursing best with my feet on the ground and my patients weighing less than ten pounds. There's nothing like a trip to make you appreciate home, sweet home.

The Tale of the Innominate War*

SCOTT WRAIGHT

Once upon a time, long ago and far away, there existed a small group of islands in the Upper Outer Quadrant of the Sebaceous Sea. These islands were called Incus, Stapes and Malleus, the names of gods revered by the natives. Collectively, they were known as the Isles of Langerhans . . .

The people who lived on the Isles of Langerhans were called the Synovials, best described in the epic book "The Last of the Synovials," by James Fenamore Cowper. They were clean, just and strong. Subject to Immunity, their King, they led a peaceful life; peaceful, that is, until the nation of Golgi declared war on them.

The Golgi were a short, ill-tempered, myopic, nasty people who reputedly carried on the practice of anabolism. They were abdominal people, the true villi of the story.

The Golgis declared war because of an "inflammatory" remark attributed to a Synovial at the D.B. & C. Conferences (something about their being S.O.B. that was taken the wrong way).

The Golgi Vesicles began the war with Coronal Sutures in charge of the invasion of the Isles of Langerhans. Meanwhile, the good people of Synovial were lying on the beach, listening to Peri Neal on the radio, drinking Pepsin, and having a good time. Suddenly they heard an announcement from their leader, General Malaise—an attack was pending, and he was calling out the Axillary. Major Surgery was indicated as leader of the Costal Defense. The Synovials were preparing for war.

Initially a navel battle was proposed, but the Synovials lacked a large force of Lymph Vessels, so they could only dig in and stay alert.

It was dawn of the following day. The Golgi's Coronal Sutures had only to wait for the high nucleotide to begin the attack.

It was a viscose attack indeed. The Golgi moved in massed peristalsis through the Canal of Schlemm—so-called because of Rear Admiral Schlemm's victorious use of anatomic bombs in Huntington's Chorea—and onward to the main island of Malleus.

The Synovials waiting on the beach were feeling pretty squamous about this time, but remained steadfast of purpose. The Golgi began firing their ships' guns, until the islands pulsated with great fibroblasts. Quickly they moved in and landed troops on the shore, led by none other than that star of stage, screen and sandy beach, Efrem Embolus Jr. The two armies began to articulate. The Synovials were being pushed back further and further in spite of the unflagging attempts of their Dorsal Planes that were bombing the Golgi by dropping great bundles of his. Their efforts seemed to be in vein.

Finally, the Golgi advance was halted on the Sagittal Plain, where a courageous Synovial soldier named Private Parts rallied his troops and set up a counter offensive.

Now the Golgi were in a real neurolemma. They were eventually surrounded and forced to surrender. As a Synovial soldier was later heard to say, "We pulled the ruga right out from under em." Homeostasis had returned. All the captured Golgi were thrown into Schwann Cells.

It is said that the sight of his surrendering army put Coronal Sutures in an aqueous humour. In any event, he took a lethal Bowman's Capsule and died of strabismus.

Major Surgery was promoted to General Surgery; Private Parts was decorated; and everyone lived happily ever after.

*Reprinted with permission from The Canadian Nurse/L'infirmiere canadienne, ©1978; 74(11):14–15.

Twas the Night Before Christmas (at PRN General)*

NANCY CORR, R.N., ET AL.

'Twas the night before Christmas and all through
the wing
The house staff was quiet, the lights didn't ring.

The patients were poseyed in bed for their rest
While visions of elephants sat on each chest.

The TED hose were hung by the chart desk with care,
In hopes that the doctors would soon show up there.

One nurse in her sweatshirt, the rest in their wraps,
Had just settled down for their forty-wink naps.

When out in the hall there arose such a clatter,
They sprang from their chairs to see what was
the matter.

Away from the desk they all flew like a flash.
The coffee went flying! (A foot found the trash!)

Then what to their wondering eyes should appear
But the nurse from ER: "Your new patient is here."

More rapid than eagles these care-givers came.
"But nobody called!" one was heard to exclaim.

The little old patient looked weakly and sick;
The wrist band he wore bore the ID "Saint Nick."

"Get lido, get lab, get O_2, he looks pale!
An IVAC, a tempspar, a gown, and the scale!

"To the end of the hall, to room 328 . . .
Let's get him admitted before it's too late!!"

He was dressed all in fur from his head to his feet;
This was promptly replaced by a gown and a sheet.

His bundle of toys someone started to clear:
"It's at your own risk if you have them kept here."

The stump of a pipe he had started to puff.
"There's oxygen on—will you stop with that stuff!"

Then a nurse grabbed his pipe and said, "Sorry,
my dear.
We *do not allow* any smoking in here."

Then he said he was hungry, this stout little fellow,
And frowned when they said, "All we have here is
Jello."

"Have you dentures?" they asked. "Any allergies,
please?
Know anyone else who has had this disease?"

"I've been toiling," he sighed, "every night in my shop.
There was so much to do that I just couldn't stop."

"Now, try to relax, dear, and get lots of rest.
You don't have to worry, for we are the best.

"If you follow instructions and do as we say,
In two or three weeks you'll be well on your way.

"Just put on your light if you need something more.
Either way we'll be back for your bath about four."

The IV above and the rails on the bed
Convinced Mr. Nick there was something to dread.

"You say I need blood tests and therefore must stay,
But I won't miss this night for the whole AMA!"

And seeing the nurses' quick looks of alarm
He gave them a wink and he turned on the charm:

"I'm sure you mean well, but this simply can't be.
There are millions of children relying on me."

So, pulling the monitor leads from his chest,
He promised them, "Dearies, tomorrow I'll rest."

Then quick as a wink he was out of the sack,
And into his clothes, with his pack on his back.

He spoke not a word, but charged straight out the door,
Down the hall toward 3 West . . . till they saw him
no more.

But they heard him exclaim as he ran out of sight:
"Merry Christmas to all, and to all a good night!"

(By the way, for those readers who still are in doubt,
His enzymes came back: An MI was ruled out.)

* Published in RN, December 1979, Vol. 42(12), pages 36–37. Copyright
©1979 Medical Economics Publishing, Montvale, N.J. Reprinted by
permission.

NURSES VS. DOCTORS

If you can remember way back into your childhood, you must have played doctor and nurse. The most vocal or male child always became "the" doctor, while the female or younger kids usually became nurses. The youngest child or the family pet always got bandaged, poked, prodded, and needled. After a brief period of tranquility, screams, arguments, and tears often drove one or more of the players to quit the game.

Those childhood games were excellent training for surviving the continuing tensions that plague both professions to this day. That bright, shiny stethoscope so fiercely fought for can be attained by each and every one. In the final analysis, all players are winners when they serve the patient's best interests.

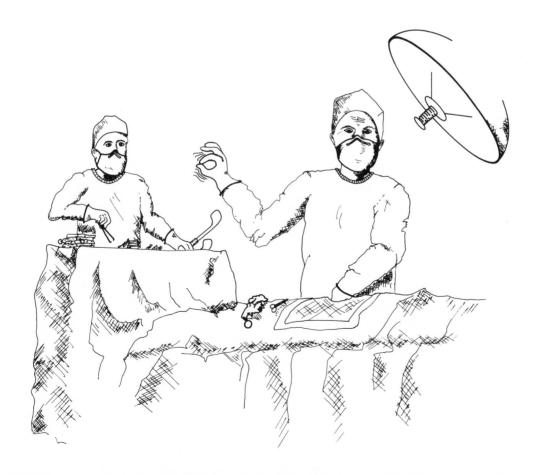

How to Drive Nurses Crazy*

and ease them out of nursing

HARVEY N. MANDELL, M.D.

Some of our colleagues seem to think they can best serve humanity by making life miserable for nurses.[†] If this was one of the goals that led you to medical school, I suggest careful reading of the following tips to help you succeed in your task.

For attending physicians: When the nurse calls you with new laboratory data, tell her to call whoever is consulting in the appropriate field and suggest she not bother you. For consultants on the same case: When the nurse calls you with new laboratory data, scold her and state emphatically that she should have called the attending physician.

Write orders illegibly and leave the floor before the nurse can get to them. When she calls for clarification, have your answering service say you are gone for the day and signed out to another doctor. If you are the other doctor, say you don't know anything about the patient.

Write most of your orders in the metric system but just enough of them in the apothecary system so nurses have to learn both. Let "g" stand for both grain and gram. Don't let your obvious obsolescence bother you.

If you are one of several physicians treating the same patient, don't look at the other doctors' orders before or after you write yours. It's okay if you order one aminoglycoside for a patient already receiving another. Let the nurse call the other doctors and try to straighten it out. Your time is much too valuable to spend it trying to avoid conflicting orders.

If you plan to be away for a few days, do not tell the head nurse. Let her find out about it when your patient is in respiratory arrest and the answering service is not sure who is covering.

Insist that only you can order an aspirin or laxative for your patients, but when you put a patient on a ventilator turn the whole thing over to the nurses and respiratory therapists. Tell them not to bother you with the details and to get arterial blood gases whenever they want. Don't confess to them that you haven't the slightest idea what the tidal volume should be.

If you are standing next to the chart rack, wait for a nurse to come by and ask her to get your patient's chart for you. If she does it, ask her to get you a pen so you can write orders. If she says she is too busy, pout. Then tell everyone that the nurses on that floor are no good.

Just as you leave the floor give one more verbal order that no one quite understands. Then forget the order. When the nurses call for clarification, suggest they pay more attention to you.

Never read nurses' notes but grumble that they never tell you anything about your patients.

Criticize nurses vigorously and publicly when they make mistakes. When you err, shrug it off and say that everyone makes mistakes.

Always go to the head of the line in the cafeteria because you have to be in the OR in five minutes. Then take 20 minutes for lunch and dawdle over your coffee for 20 more.

When a nurse calls you at 6 AM about your patient's deteriorating condition, state firmly that she could have waited until 8 o'clock to tell you. Then come in at 7:30 AM and order everything stat. Question why everything is not ready for you.

After changing the dressing over an infected wound, drop the old dressing on the floor. Don't wash your hands before attending your next patient. Make it clear that hand washing and sterile technique are for others.

If you're not sure whether your patient should be restrained, write the vague order, "Restrain patient prn." If the family complains that Granny is restrained, say the nurses showed poor judgment. If the family finds Granny on the floor next to the bed with a

*Reprinted from Postgraduate Medicine, ©1983; 73(3):30 with permission from McGraw-Hill, Inc. and the author.

[†]I am speaking here of stereotypical male physicians who often treat female nurses somewhat differently than they treat male nurses.

broken hip, say the nurses showed poor judgment. Later, explain that "prn" means the nurse should restrain the patient three minutes before the patient plans to climb over the side rails and break her hip.

Tell your patient she is going home Tuesday but tell the charge nurse you plan to discharge Wednesday. This keeps everyone off guard.

Write preop surgical prep orders for lumbar spine when you really mean cervical spine. Act betrayed when the patient comes to the OR with neck unprepped.

Don't return nurses' telephone calls for orders. You are much too busy to do that. Later, raise a fuss because your patient received no medication for pain.

If the nurses make coffee on the ward, help yourself to it but never contribute to the coffee fund. Nurses' incomes are about the same as doctors', so they enjoy providing these small services.

Never carry a dressing tray, for a surgeon's hands are precious. Have the nurse do it.

Never help a nurse reposition a patient in bed; she should be strong enough to do it by herself.

In surgery, if a liter of unexpected and unwanted arterial blood suddenly obscures your operative field, immediately blame the scrub nurse for not having the proper setup and the circulating nurse for not acting quickly enough to get someone to bail you out. When panic subsides, restrain yourself from thanking them for their help.

If you're hungry and you see a nurse's lunch in the refrigerator, take some of it. She probably had you in mind when she prepared it.

Finally, if your patient's family asks you to tell the nurses how much they appreciate the good nursing care Grandpa received, forget to relay the message.

Editor's note: The response to Dr. Mandell's article is "How to Drive Doctors Crazy and Ease Them into Malpractice Suits" by Janice L. Dennis, Postgraduate Medicine, 1983; 73(6):303–304.

Spare the Fools
and Interns*

THOM SCHWARZ, R.N.

He'll show up in your hospital in July. His pockets will bulge with a shiny new stethoscope, ophthalmoscope, reflex hammer, calculator, diagnostic manuals, and pens; and he'll have a PDR under his arm. His white jacket will be as immaculate as a headwaiter's, and the grin on his ID card photo would shame a Cheshire cat. He'll look like a cross between the ultimately-prepared boy scout and a sacrificial lamb. He's just one of the upcoming crop of interns, fresh out of school and ready to play his comic/tragic role like a modern-day Charlie Chaplin.

If you're fortunate, he'll have come from a program that emphasizes hands-on time with patients. But if your luck has run out, you could have a severe problem on your hands: someone who's inept, clumsy, and fearful; who doesn't know enough to step out of the way when the patient retches. The temptation to ridicule him seems irresistible. Yet this is the very moment when we should be doing just the opposite, not just for his sake, but for the patient's—and our own.

I've watched his counterparts for many years. The last time I encountered one of these fledglings was in a large teaching hospital in New York City. A veteran of several years in other hospitals, I already knew what to expect when the "tern" (a derisive nickname) arrived. But he wasn't beaming with MD self-confidence and smugness, and he didn't show the remotest hint of the MD self-righteousness that irritates legions of nurses every day. I think he felt every bit as ridiculous as he looked. He knew he was not fully prepared for what was to come.

His family had heaped praise upon him since the day he announced his medical school intentions. His patients would view him as residing among the heavenly anointed—far above the angels in white. He had a degree from a fine university and had been accepted into a good medical program. But his $50,000 education

had been full of clinical holes. He couldn't give an injection, pass a nasogastric tube, or even take an accurate blood pressure.

Full of academic knowledge rather than basic technical skills, he was one of these interns who had somehow missed even the most prosaic pearl of hospital lore. He was hesitant to approach and touch patients and didn't know how to take leave gracefully. It's difficult to examine a patient at arm's length, but he tried. And he never thought to replace the sheet over the naked patient after examining him.

Later, his senior residents would gleefully watch him painfully master each task and procedure while offering minimal assistance and encouragement, often at the expense of the patient's comfort. A junior resident explained his non-help attitude: "I had to suffer through it all, so now he's going to have to go through it all, too."

So, it was not surprising that, within a few weeks, the intern was physically and psychologically—much like a new nursing grad—totally exhausted, numbed by the inhuman workload, isolated, lonely, and fast becoming inured to the pain of others.

Trying Not to Feel Disdainful

The temptation is strong for nurses to vent pent-up resentments on such a hapless intern in reparation for all the years of abuse suffered at the hands of obnoxious attendings. And, if you assume that this same intern will someday hatch into a boorish MD himself, the urge to get your licks in while you can may almost seem justified. I must confess that, with this particular intern, the thought did cross my mind. How much fun it would have been to bait him in a game of medical, psychological, and clinical one-upmanship that I knew I couldn't lose at this stage of his training!

*Published in RN, June 1982, Vol. 75(6), pages 40–41. Copyright ©1982 Medical Economics Publishing, Montvale, N.J. Reprinted by permission.

But there were good reasons for resisting this urge. An MD after his name doesn't automatically make someone obnoxious. In fact, it turns only a small minority sour. So to punish an intern in advance just doesn't make sense. Nor does a nurse who howls with laughter when an intern bungles patient care present either him or the patient with a particularly sterling example of a caring, sensitive health care practitioner. Maybe he *is* the most hilariously bumbling beginner you've ever seen. And there may be time later to recount his ineptness in private, perhaps even share it with him. But when you're in front of the patient, it's time to close ranks as health care professionals and preserve the intern's dignity, to say nothing of helping the patient to trust in his care.

Teaching the Fledgling to Fly

I recall a particular morning in the emergency room, when I was still fairly close to being a rookie on the staff myself. I raised my cup to the intern and greeted him with a cheery, "What's up, Doc?" He could only smile crookedly as a junior resident laughed, "He's not a doc; he's only a 'tern.'" The other residents and some nurses joined the chorus of giggles while the senior residents smiled in silent acquiescence.

As if this were not demeaning enough, the same junior resident later called the intern to admit a "bag lady" from the streets who was suffering from a plethora of chronic complaints. Standing at the foot of the stretcher, he pointed at the pitiful patient and announced loudly to the intern, "This is just the sort of patient for you. Not so sick that you might hurt her, but filthy enough to make you gag." This treatment went on until the intern learned how to avoid the "hazing." But treating urban, homeless indigents as non-persons is a nasty business—not a tradition to be encouraged

in newcomers who might someday use it to vent their own frustrations.

Nurses and residents can quickly forget experiences gathered at the bottom of the clinical totem pole. I made a resolution not to, deciding instead, to help facilitate this intern's transition to clinical practice in any way I could. I quietly talked him through procedures, passed on time-saving tips, and whispered words of encouragement when he failed or mastered a skill. My reasons were not entirely altruistic. I was offering him some kindness and respect, it's true; but I was also hoping this might be passed on to the patients—or even to other nurses.

I later discovered other nurses who had taken on the same job: showing interns some basic nursing skills and teaching them how to view patients as people with health care and related problems, not as medical aberrations or lab animals. We possess what many interns desperately need and desire: practical clinical expertise and good common sense in dealing with patients. It's not really our job, and it takes plenty of tact and patience, but we can teach these interns some really important lessons—even if the oral tradition of their seniors, and perhaps their own pride, prevent them from openly seeking help and friendship.

There's a possibility, of course, that our best efforts will go for naught. There will always be interns who revert to insensitive treatment of patients or to the sexist tradition of taking the nurse for granted and bypassing her as a teacher and friend. And we will never be without those who benefit from our concern but refuse to give due recognition. That's hardly the point, though. It's this kind of caring that made us nurses, and it's this kind of professionalism in caring that shows we made it.

Show *that* to some beleaguered intern.

Gown Tiers I Have Known*

B. S. CRAWFORD, M.B., F.R.C.S.

Among other things my scraggy neck houses a prominent and tender larynx. For some unexplained reason it has been the target for destruction by various members of what was once called the fair sex. Their weapon is the modern equivalent of the garrotte and it takes the form of a thong-like band concealed in the upper edge of each operating gown. The attacker approaches from the rear and manipulates the weapon holding one of the top tapes in each hand. An expert uses a number of ploys, for example a combination of a backward pull, elevation on the larynx and rapid saw-like action which together can be effective, yes even devastating. The application of the right amount of slice and follow-through produces a nasty laryngeal injury, and with care the victim's cry can be stifled at source. A true expert can cause a "lovely" cardiac arrest by adding a nifty clobber on the vagus, but unfortunately this merciful end to a promising surgical career is rare.

I am a self-styled authority on operating gowns. Man and boy I must have worn over 15,000, but only one at a time. If they were folded and stacked they would fill a very large space such as an administrator's office, or twenty-five surgeon's rooms. In my long hours of vigil spent waiting for anaesthetists I have had ample time to ponder over the problem and I now believe that there are three main faults—and a possible solution.

Faults

1. Me

I should retire and stoke the boilers. Alternatively I should wear a dog-collar of suitable material or have my larynx excised—this would solve two problems at once.

2. Gown Tiers

They come in many varieties and the experienced surgeon can spot them as they emerge from the sluice. In order not to bore you stiff I shall only describe three.

(a) Farmers' Daughters   They have big bones, Suffolk Punch ankles and bags of enthusiasm. They are adept at harnessing horses and tackle this gown-tying lark with the same verve. The laryngeal haematomas they produce are made to last and are guaranteed to silence all victims for a week. Not only do these Amazons grasp the tapes with energy, they finish the job with a nice flourish to test whether the old man has anything left in him—this is the B.H.T. or bottom hem tug well loved by mothers dispatching little ones to school and designed to remind them Who is Boss. If it is well applied the force can fracture a clavicle and shake the whole frame which serves to take the pain away from the larynx.

(b) The Diminutive Type   These bright-eyed undersized professionals tackle the job with the zeal of mountaineers. They leap up to catch the top tapes and then hang on for dear life, inserting one of their clogs into a convenient clog-hole such as the popliteal space, while they inflict a laryngeal injury worthy of the great Kung Fu. In every gown-tier's little suitcase is an Administrator's clip-board so I must stifle all criticism and get tied up in the knees bend position; otherwise I certainly will end up stoking the boilers.

(c) The Seductive Type   A whiff of Chanel No. 1 announces her stealthy arrival. She starts by searching for the third tape down and many a young surgeon has felt a tiny warm hand fumbling in his R.I.F. She wears a crucifix dangling in the intermammary cleft thereby contravening Circular SB/109/A/424/76. Beware, because she is a deadly strangler who ties the top tape *last* once the victim has been seduced. (Praying Mantis type.)

3. The Gown

I have never been impressed by the standard of surgeon's wear. I believe that a man will live on the moon before a satisfactory outfit is produced. I venture to

* Reprinted with permission from NATNews: The British Journal of Theatre Nursing, ©1984; 21(12):20.

suggest a modification which will fall on deaf ears to enter closed minds.

The Solution

(i) If the top tapes are shifted downwards about 4 cm, tension will be transferred from the sharp upper edge of the gown to the broad acres across the sternum. This will solve the problem in males—and in some females.

(ii) All nurses will have to pass the D.G.T. (Diploma of Gown Tying) until this modification is implemented (F.N.C./741/88A/77).

I cannot understand why nurses say I am sarcastic. I remember with gratitude and affection all who have tied and occasionally untied my gowns in the past and the thought brings a tear to my eye and a lump in the throat.

Gown Wearers I Have Known*

Reply to B. S. Crawford, M.B., F.R.C.S.

F. WHEELER, S.R.N.

Recently I watched a very small nurse struggle to "take" a total hip replacement operation. This event confirmed my belief that to be tall is an asset for a theatre nurse especially when "tying in" surgeons.

This apparently elementary task can be quite a daunting procedure fraught with hazards. Surgeons who appear at ward rounds smiling at patients and charming to sister, take on a different character once they enter the operating theatre. Any experienced theatre nurse can recognize them before the swing doors have banged shut. Seeing Mr. X in revealing theatre garb instead of the familiar pin-stripe is quite off-putting. Hairy ears, bow-legs, scraggy necks and portly waistlines are now apparent, but scrubbing-up is the real give away indicating what the theatre staff are in for. Having height and a fair reach certainly helps to deal with medical friends!

TYPE 1 The Gabbler crashes through the doors calling out greetings to all and sundry to announce his arrival. Scrub solution is splashed everywhere and dripped all across the theatre floor whilst he walks to and fro talking to theatre staff and the scrub nurse in the laying-up room.

Tying up his gown is not easy as he continues to turn around, walk about and issue further requests. It is equally difficult to resist the urge to issue the command "stay" in the true Woodhouse fashion. Having stepped back on nurse's toes, ripped, dropped his gloves, gown or both, he eventually makes it to the table leaving a trail of debris and an exhausted gown-tier behind him!

TYPE 2 Can be described as **Macho**. Scrubbing-up is conducted slowly to give all the chance to view his strong muscular hands and forearms. Donning the gown is also performed with care to demonstrate the full width of shoulders and torso. A deep-throated request not to tie the tapes too tight will be followed by further flexing of muscles just to prove the point. Front ties are held wide to allow a final show of profile before striding away.

TYPE 3 In contrast there is the **Fastidious** type. The procedure of scrubbing and gowning up begins with a close inspection of nails and hands, accompanied by a frown or smile depending on the state of same. Brushes that are too stiff have to be changed and taps are carefully adjusted to give the correct flow and

*Reprinted with permission from NATNews: The British Journal of Theatre Nursing, ©1985; 22(3):10.

temperature of water. Washing is carefully carried out to the allotted time and drying materials dropped from shoulder height to prevent contamination. The tier-in is worried and warned "mind my neck," which happens to be a feature that only an Aberdeen Angus steer would be proud of!

Front ties are held very wide making the grasping of them difficult and instruction is usually given as to their required tension! Tiers-in must resist the temptation to wrench them together with full force but comply with a smile and step back with a sigh.

Faults

Gone is the surgeon who appears to understand why he scrubs up and how to accomplish it correctly.

Solution

All medical students should be instructed on the procedure before being allowed within the hallowed walls!

All theatre nurses should be shown how to "tie in" with consideration to the wearer.

The Gown

As usual it is assumed that the Lunar occupier is male, but if this dominance gave way to those who appreciate fabrics, materials and most importantly design, this garment could be made more comfortable and acceptable.

Solution

I refer not to fashion and couture but the ones who really know about clothes—those who design and sew for children. Every mother knows the raglan sleeve (his Lordship proved it) is easier to put on than the set-in variety and much easier to press. Tapes and ties could be replaced by Velcro strips either across or down the length of the back opening making the front tie obsolete. The mandarin collar (the stand up bit) is unnecessary and costly to manufacture and launder. The raglan design could be sloped up toward the neck in one piece, making surgeon garotting difficult—what a pity!

How practical to have a variety of sizes. In my theatre the standard gown has to fit a 6 ft. 3 in. surgeon and a 4 ft. 11 in. nurse—not at the same time of course! But maybe this situation could be altered if the designers, makers, buyers and launderers would take notice of the wearers and tiers.

Conclusion

So having height and reach has been a definite advantage in coping with many gown wearers over the years. All those times with trolley laid, instruments set and sutures mounted waiting for the "emergency" operation to commence has given me plenty of opportunity for observation of gown wearers.

Perhaps it's time I put these advantages to better use and headed for the boiler house if it's not already overstaffed.

Humor in the OR*

JOEL H. GOLDBERG

There's always somebody who never sees the lighter side of an environment as serious as the operating room ("My surroundings are not very funny," notes one nurse) or who thinks humor there is never appropriate ("I do not allow funny incidents," grumbles one chief of surgery).

Still, there are plenty of chuckles—judging by the surprisingly large number of anecdotes in our survey about scrub pants falling to a surgeon's ankles, and the number of chief surgeons appearing in a dress because no pants were available.

Humor in the OR usually happens spontaneously, and often you have to have been there or know the players personally to appreciate it. Some of it involves black humor, as might be expected in a life-or-death situation. Some of it is classic slapstick. In any case, here are incidents that some of our survey respondents considered "the funniest thing they'd ever seen happen in the OR":

From a Kentucky orthopedist: "I told a new circulating nurse I needed an Otis elevator and she went to central supply for it." (A popular variation is sending the new nurse for "another box of fallopian tubes.")

From a Nevada neurosurgeon: "As he proceeded with an operation, a colleague kept complaining that the OR's air conditioning was on too strong. When he finally stepped from the table, he tripped over his scrub pants because they'd dropped to his ankles at the start of the procedure."

From a general surgeon: "The anesthetized patient reached up into the field to retract his own wound."

From an Illinois thoracic surgeon: "One doctor who works with me always wears his glasses perched on the end of his nose. One day during surgery they fell into the abdominal cavity."

In New York, about to undergo a hernia repair, a middle-aged man had been administered pentothal—but apparently wasn't very deep yet. So when the surgeon began to swab the operative site with a Betadine-soaked sponge, the patient stirred. "Oh, Maria—No!" he moaned. "Stop it! I'm sleeping!"

An orthopedist in Wisconsin recalls the time "the patient arrested on the table. I looked quickly at the anesthesiologist, who promptly yelled out, 'Call 911!'"

A general surgeon in Minnesota had trouble stifling a smile the day his chief of surgery "slipped and fell butt first into the kick bucket." (An RN at another hospital tells of an angry surgeon kicking a kick bucket across the room, and an equally angry scrub nurse booting it right back.)

Before being put to sleep for a procedure, a patient at a hospital in Kansas was being questioned by the surgeon about a history of chest pain. "Yes," he replied. "Occasionally I have some vagina pain on the upper left side."

Misunderstandings are frequent: A Virginia nurse recalls a patient having a hernia repair. When the surgeon told the patient to strain, he thought the surgeon had said "scream." "So he did," she says. "We had to pull the entire team off the ceiling. Now that surgeon tells hernia patients to bear down."

And a doctor in Arizona recalls the time shortly after a cholecystectomy, that a nurse delivered the gallstones to the patient—the usual custom—in a clean, plastic vial: "The nurse said, 'Here they are for you,' and the patient popped them in his mouth and swallowed them all."

From a nurse in California: "The assistant surgeon's pants fell while he was scrubbed, exposing the cutest boxer shorts with red hearts on them." (A nurse in

Virginia describes a nearly identical incident—except that the surgeon wasn't wearing *any* shorts.)

Patients quip frequently. In Maryland, a patient was undergoing a vasectomy when a 4-by-4 pad caught fire. Everybody remained calm. As we put the flames out, the patient lifted his head and asked, "Are we roasting marshmallows?" In Oklahoma, a shooting victim was brought to the OR for removal of a foreign body—the bullet had hit loose change in his pants pocket, and pieces of the coins were imbedded in his leg. The patient pondered the gowned and masked surgeon, and remarked, "Well, I guess it's only normal to wear a mask when taking someone's money."

At a hospital in Indiana, one woman inspired a chuckle even while under anesthesia. She was having a frozen-section breast biopsy, and the surgery team found a note taped to her right breast reading. "Smile—you're on 'Candid Camera.'"

So You Want to Work in the O.R.*

KAREN M. JORDAN, C.S.T.

You've decided you want to work in the operating room. I hate to do this, but there are a few things you should know before you begin. You've heard it's so rewarding—receiving the gratitude of patients and the admiration of doctors. And it's so educational—working with intelligent, dedicated doctors with years of training behind them.

It is true, the knowledge the surgeons exhibit is amazing. But let's face it—in the quest for a degree—some areas received little, if any, attention. One of the main areas of neglect is the ability to tell or estimate time. When surgeons are asked how much longer it will take to finish a procedure, a basic deficiency rolls in like a clap of thunder. In dealing with this, one formula that works quite well is to double the time estimate and add 37 minutes. This formula works well also when they call to estimate time of arrival to begin a case. Sometimes it works better to triple the time and add 49 minutes—it depends on the surgeon. You're probably already familiar with this weakness from having spent hours in a doctor's waiting room.

There's another problem. I'm sure many patients would jump off the operating table and run if they were aware of it. A surgeon comes into the room, scrubbed, ready to begin the operation. After drying hands on a cloth towel, some surgeons stand before the containers—one a cloth laundry bag and one a plastic hamper liner—and try to decide where the towel goes. We generally try to let them work it out for themselves, but the patient is anesthetized and we have to set a time limit.

After being gowned and gloved, we hand our surgeons another towel to wipe gloves. Now we're back to step one. Some surgeons attempt to cover their confusion by pretending they're Magic Johnson going for a long shot. They trot across the room, turn and let the towel fly. When it drops two feet from the containers, the decision is out of their hands.

We've been using disposable drapes that have a large white piece of paper over the fenestration with the words "REMOVE PRIOR TO USE." One can only believe that some didn't. I've heard surgeons explain that it's there for legal reasons. It's best to just nod in agreement—with a mask on they can't see the smile on your face.

It's so dramatic working as a team member "saving lives and curing the ills of humanity!" Don't be fooled. Some days don't quite reach those heights. The first months in the OR are unbelievable until you realize

* Reprinted from Point of View, ©1986; 23(2):20–21 with permission from Ethicon, Inc. Edited from the original.

that magnitude of the situation is not always the prime consideration. Take it with a grain of salt when you're told, "This is the worst fracture I've ever seen": "I've never operated on a hotter appendix (or gallbladder)"; "That's the biggest ulcer I've ever seen—it's a wonder he's alive"; "I've only seen a deformity this bad once before"; "These adhesions are like concrete," *ad infinitum*. There will be days when you'll be involved with a small hernia, an atrophied uterus, a normal appendix, and a boring arthroscopy. And you'll love the boredom. It could be worse. It's difficult to be fascinated with any procedure that lasts more than six hours. And any operation that begins after midnight lacks a lot of the beauty and wonder that would have been present 12 hours before. But at least you're well trained and ready to face the challenge.

Trust me when I tell you that you're going to believe you're marginally retarded, or worse, long before assurance arrives. I know. Once I spent quite some time in an instrument room searching before I went back and announced that I couldn't find the plastic scissors— all I found were metal. A friend of mine was told by a surgeon to "point" a suture. Never having heard this expression, rather than put a hemostat on the suture, she asked him, "Which direction?"

Expressions indigenous to medicine can be a challenge. I can remember how appalled I was to hear tissue described as friable. Why not broilable or sautéable? During a particularly trying procedure, a surgeon who strikes terror in the hearts of the most seasoned OR personnel asked me for the "dulox"—he needed it NOW! In my panic, all I could think of was to wonder why he needed a laxative. I had never heard that expression before.

Hand signals can be an efficient way to make wants and needs known. But not all signalers follow the standardized movements. Attempting to decipher the code keeps you on your toes, as does trying to understand a mumbler. Mumblers speak like normal human beings when you're visiting with them in the lounge. But let them tie a mask over their face and suddenly all the separate letters that make words combine into a long, completely unintelligible utterance. Once this happens, it's as if they don't want you to be aware of their problem so they lower their voices and bow their heads. You have to learn to pick up on sounds and attempt to relate them to words that would fit at that stage of the operation. An "s" sound mumbled at one point would probably mean saline; at another point it might be suture. Experience helps.

You must think I've become very cynical. I prefer to think of life in the OR as realistic. The surgeons and staff members are human beings—some more so than others! I've worked in the OR for ten plus years, so I've wiped some of the stars out of my eyes. But I still love to come to work.

Communicating with Surgeons, Once You Learn the Language, Is Possible Most of the Time*

PATTY SWENSON, R.N.

"Communicating in the OR is difficult." Too right and amen. The reason for this and the blame (if there be blame) can be directly traced to the fact that most OR nurses sign on with only their mother tongue as a means of communication. Although the job descriptions never mention it, fluency in "Surgeon Speak" and its several dialects—one for each surgeon—is easily the key to on-the-job success or failure.

For example, the manufacturer's catalog will refer, and correctly so, to a certain instrument as a Mayo clamp, but only a fool will ever expect to hear it called by that name. Instead surgeons will ask for heavy curves, curved sixes, fat Kellys, and in moments of intense concentration, "that one over there." Kitners, kuntners, peanuts, and occasionally, cherries, all refer to the same blunt dissector. Schnitz, snits, and tonsils are the same stroke to different folk. A ribbon is a malleable is a flat bendable.

One surgeon will call an instrument by many pet names, depending upon how it will be used. Alone it's a right angle; feed a piece of suture into its little beak and you have a tie on a Mixter. The list is endless, and I will bet there are some regional variations that would bring tears to my eyes.

But conversation in the OR is less than stimulating, despite the occasional burst of confusion from instrument names. Most of the exchanges are hardly enough to keep the mind alive. I quote:

"Give me a tie."
"What kind?"
"Any kind."
"Here's 3-0 silk."
"Terrific!"
"You're welcome."
"I didn't ask for a rope. I asked for a tie."

"You have it."
"Then what is THIS?"
"Three-0 silk."
"Man oh man. This sure doesn't FEEL like 3-0."
"What DOES it feel like?"
"It feels like 2-0."
"Trust me."
"I TRUST you. But next time I want thin 3-0."
"Ooookay."

Surgeon Signal

Next we have "Surgeon Signal." This is a series of hand signals substituted for the spoken word, used to request objects with perfectly good given names. They are used instead because: (a) the surgeon in question doesn't know the real name, (b) is saving his voice for bigger and better things, (c) assumes the scrub nurse is deaf, or (d) all of the above.

Among the more common signals are
- the forefinger and middle finger moving up and down against each other in a scissors-like fashion meaning, "I wish to cut."
- the thumb and forefinger meeting one another in a rapid pinching motion usually indicating the desire for a pickup or is a sure sign of burnout.
- the hand formed into a semi-fist, whipped rapidly in a partially clockwise direction, quaintly requesting a needle and thread on a needle holder. Now really, wouldn't the simple use of the word suture be a lot less wearing on everyone?

One of my favorite surgeons has a habit of simply holding out his hand, as if to make a left-hand turn,

*Adapted from the AORN Journal, Vol. 40, p 784–785, November, 1984, with permission. Copyright © AORN Inc., 10170 East Mississippi Avenue, Denver, CO 80231.

giving you the option of placing in it whatever you think will strike his fancy.

Surgeon Snag

To me, the average surgeon's concept of time is the eighth wonder of the world and something for which there is no rational explanation. "Surgeon time" is not necessarily "clock time" as I know it. There is no established rule for converting one to the other, but a safe guideline is if your surgeon says, "This will only take 45 minutes, " DOUBLE it! In many cases—and these you quickly become familiar with or go mad—TRIPLING it is a more realistic approach to estimating when the room will be available for someone else. No matter what *they* say, *you* know better. And *they* know *you* know. And *you* know *they* know *you* know. Which is 75% of the reason for the half-crazed expressions worn by surgery supervisors during working hours and why they are so often observed babbling pathetically to no one in particular.

The remaining 25% of the cause contributing to the downfall of even the brightest and best OR supervisor is directly traceable to the "Supply and Demand Equation." This boils down to something like, "The number of supplies and instruments a surgeon says he will need is inversely proportionate to the amount he will ultimately require." This law is most effective after 3 pm and on weekends.

Most surgeons manage to stay reasonably calm and collected under the most trying circumstances. But now and then the rare individual comes along who communicates mainly by tantrum and is directly responsible for the percentage of OR nurses eagerly pouring their pathetic tales of woe into the nearest crisis hotline. This character doesn't enter a room—he lays siege to it, causing the barometer to automatically drop three points. The moment anything displeases him (usually within the first 20 seconds), he is capable of throwing a tantrum that makes Ivan the Terrible look like a pussycat. His ritual of impatience can begin with an erratic tapping of one or both feet followed by a seizure-like rolling of the eyes. Once he is into the swing of things you will hear him gnashing his teeth on every other beat. Soon the rhythm section is joined by a vocal rendition of deep, heart-rending sounds which you can safely assume are sighs . . . or maybe even sobs . . . depending upon how badly he is being abused. On a really good day, and without missing a beat, he will manage to gravitate away from the table toward the nearest wall where he will take several deep breaths in a supreme effort to regain his immaculate composure. Thus fortified, he is ready to once again cope with the stupidity that surrounds him, "black as a pit from pole to pole."

But I repeat—this type is the exception rather than the rule, so the number of deserving surgeons eliminated by homicidal nurses remains relatively static from year to year.

All in all, after years of research, observation, and personal experience, I can safely say that communicating with surgeons, once you learn the language and establish a few ground rules, is possible most of the time.

WATCH YOUR LANGUAGE

Communication in all its various forms is the core of all human behavior. Each profession has its own specialized vocabulary that defines members of the group. Learning that special language used between nurses, coworkers, patients, and physicians is essential to providing quality nursing care.

Effective communication in a practicing profession such as nursing is a combination of seeing, listening, and feeling. Illegible handwriting and the liberal use of jargon, acronyms, and "medspeak" are often the root causes of confusion. Though such errors can be funny, they can also be fatal.

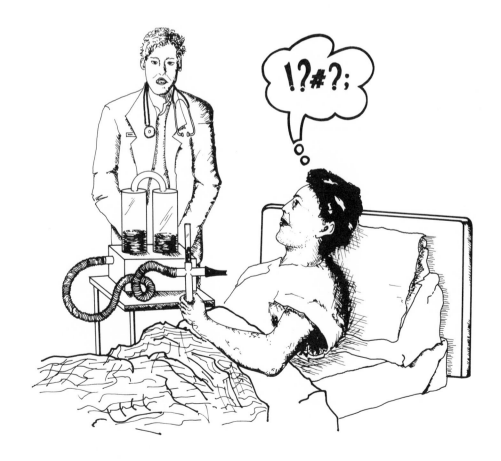

Acute, Fulminating Jargonitis*

ELLEN GOLDENSOHN

Take the case of Susan P, a 29-year-old R.N.. In infancy and early childhood, she had a normal history. She spoke her first word at twelve months and was able to write her own name by the age of four. During her school days, she spoke and wrote plainly, and was clearly understood by her parents and classmates. Through secondary school and most of her nursing education, she progressed normally in written and oral expression in the English language. In some classes, say her professors, she excelled. It was only after several years of clinical experience, in the midst of preparing an article for a professional journal, that she was found to be suffering from acute, fulminating jargonitis. Probable cause? Overexposure to the writings of government bureaucrats and academics, as well as lowered resistance to carriers in the behavioral and social sciences.

Early detection and excellent follow-up led to a complete cure for Susan, but for many other health care professionals, the disease often becomes chronic and intractable. If you're beginning to do some writing of your own and you want to avoid jargonitis, simply watch out for the following signs and symptoms. You can keep the disease from becoming serious as long as you're vigilant.

Loss of Basic Verbs

Jargonitis usually has an imperceptible onset, but the disappearance of simple Anglo-Saxon verbs is often a sign that the disease is in the early stages. Examine your manuscript carefully. If you find that you are utilizing, facilitating, implementing, and optimizing instead of merely using, helping, doing, and making the best of things, you may want to refresh your prose with a few old-fashioned monosyllables.

Be strict with yourself: Only if you can honestly say that it is more blessed to utilize than to use can you permit yourself the fancier word.

*Reprinted from Nursing Outlook, ©1982; 30(9):541 with permission from Mosby-Year Book, Inc.

Noun Chains and Noun Clusters

The appearance of noun chains is almost always a sign that jargonitis has taken hold of the host. At first, nouns may appear in seemingly innocuous pairs (*health behaviors, communication facilitation, intimacy skills*). Soon afterward, clusters appear (*health maintenance techniques, support system network*). Use of adjectives becomes sporadic; prepositional phrases are rarities. Finally, indiscriminate chains of nouns take over whole sentences: "Communication facilitation skills development intervention," writes the jargonitis sufferer. The disease has reached an acute stage and should be treated aggressively.

Loss of Direct and Indirect Objects
(Gestalt Workshop Syndrome)

This final stage is marked by the appearance of interrupted verbs. The writer creates sentences in which people *cope, share,* and *relate.* Cope with what? Share what? Relate to whom? But the reader inquires in vain; the writer believes that the reader can cope.

Treatment and Cure

Remember that nurse-writers aren't fundamentally different from any other writers. Whether you're reporting the results of a randomized controlled study on the effectiveness of nurse-midwives, describing the invasion of the Falkland Islands, or just writing a letter to your Aunt Tillie, the principles are the same. Keep your reader in mind. She or he is probably a person very much like you. Most people don't want to hack their way through a jungle of dense verbiage, but they appreciate any technical term that has a precise meaning.

In fact, technical words are fine when you're writing to an audience of peers. The terms *intubate, arteriotomy,* and *supraventricular arrhythmia* have concrete meanings for which there are no ready equivalents in day-to-day speech. As a general rule, however, don't use the technical word unless you're persuaded that it gives the reader more precise information than the common term. In other words, don't succumb to the temptation to ambulate when you can walk.

Often jargon is simply the writer's easy way out of a difficult situation. It's just so much *easier* to write that a nursing intervention positively impacts health status than it is to explain to the reader that a specific action had a specific result.

So don't resort to jargon just because you're a bit too tired to find the word that's just right. Nobody ever said that writing was easy. The truth is, a simple, readable article usually goes through more revisions than the one that seems so complicated and scholarly— and incomprehensible.

There are rewards for resisting jargonitis. Not only will journal editors more readily accept your paper for publication, but when it finally is published, people will read it. What's more, they'll understand it. So if you feel an irresistible craving to use jargon, implement the appropriate prophylactic interventions to optimize and enhance your verbalization utilization skill. Don't give in. Remember, better red than erythematous.

Nurses, Nuances, and Non-Communication: A Humorous Look at Language*

RICHARD M. GRIMES, Ph.D.
RONALD J. LORIMOR, Ph.D.

Do you occasionally wonder if you're getting through to others on the health care administration team? Do you find discussion of the same issue still results in miscommunication? We propose some of the misunderstanding results from nurses generally operating on the basis of a word's commonly understood meaning while others tend to understand nuances of meaning. To facilitate the conduct of hospital operations, we offer the following communication guide:

Afternoon Shift: A period of time when hardly anything important happens. This is proved by syllogistic logic. Only administrators do important things. Administrators are present for only a small portion of the afternoon shift. Ergo, hardly anything important happens during this time.

Average Length of Stay: A mathematical calculation which all health care administrators are dedicated to make as small as possible. However, it causes panic in the same people whenever it moves in even a modest way toward zero.

Budget: An ironclad plan for future expenditures which can only be changed at the whim of the administrator or the demand of a powerful physician.

Cost of Patient Care: A term which is synonymous with charges when discussing care for the indigent, is always too high when discussing staffing of the nursing department, and is really unknown when it is necessary for making a decision.

DRG: 1. Diagnosis Related Group. 2. A shorthand description of the government payment system which rewards those who shortchange patients and punishes

*Reprinted from Journal of Nursing Administration, ©1989; 19(9): 22,28 with permission from J. B. Lippincott Company.

those who do otherwise. 3. A shorthand description of the government payment system which rewards the efficient and punishes those who are not. 4. A shorthand description of the government payment system which is extremely flexible in the interpretation of its effect. It therefore can be used to explain any number of management failures and decisions which leads to its being called—5. *D*amned *R*egulations of the *G*overnment.

Food Temperature: The root cause of hundreds of hours of committee meetings which are devoted to discussing whether nursing or dietary should deliver trays to patient rooms. This is usually resolved with Solomon-like wisdom by deciding on one or the other and reversing the decision on an annual basis.

Night Shift: A period of time when nothing important happens. See afternoon shift for further explanation.

Health Care Crisis: A term used to describe the state of the health care industry. This term is apparently used without regard to the state of the industry in that it has been used consistently for a half century, most of which period is also described as the "good old days."

Nursing: The department employing highly specialized professionals on weekdays between 7 and 5 o'clock. At other times, nurses undergo a marvelous transformation which makes them into pharmacists, medical records librarians, linen room managers, diagnosticians, therapists of all kinds, janitors, maids, food service workers, administrators, security guards, etc. Fortunately for the employment prospects of other health care workers, nursing's high degree of specialization returns with daylight and weekdays.

Nursing Salaries: A key element of hospital cost which must be controlled at present levels unless the hospital plans to use agency nurses. These latter salaries must be twice the rate of presently employed nurses. In exceptional circumstances, good management requires them to be three times as high.

Product Line Management: A term which is used to support the delusion that hospital administrators have control over which patients will be admitted to the hospital and what services will be ordered for them. If pursued far enough, this kind of thinking will create the ideal hospital in the administrator's mind—one with no physicians.

Prospective Payment: A reimbursement mechanism which miraculously changed laboratory, x-ray, and pharmacy from revenue centers to cost centers.

Weekends: See night shift.

"The Password, Please"*

SUSAN MOORE, R.N., B.S.N., C.C.R.N., C.E.N.

Aren't we the ones when it comes to abbreviations and special terms? We belong to a special club indeed and the only way to gain entry is to know the secret passwords. Initially, there is the general health care club. You need to know secret passwords such as "prn" and "STAT" and "BUN" to gain access. Then we have our very own exclusive club of emergency care. Lest you doubt it, just try to find out the MOI without knowing about GSWs, MVAs, T-bones, and autopeds. In some areas, it gets even more exclusive than that. One enters a whole new world when prehospital personnel talk in tens. "We're 10-23 on a 10-50 with a 10-96 and an ETA of 10. 10-4?"

Our jargon saves us time, I think. And maybe it describes things more specifically. Maybe. There is not a nurse alive who has not wasted precious time searching for a physician who wrote in passwords from another exclusive club: "illegible doctor-eze." This club is so exclusive that even the person who wrote the instructions frequently cannot interpret them. And even if they can be read, there is no guarantee they will be understood. Pity the poor patient with a head injury whose physician writes out the following discharge instructions: "If HA or LOC, F/U c̄ PMD ASAP." Certainly will, doctor.

And pharmacists! They must be clairvoyant. I have a fairly good idea of what the prescription must be because I know the patient and what the trouble is. All the pharmacist sees is a little white paper with wiggly lines on it. I am very impressed that patients aren't killed everyday by improperly filled prescriptions.

Some of our passwords are not very polite. I must admit that I have written SOB many times and at least once in my life I have fully intended both meanings. And we can't omit GOMER, immortalized in *House of God*. Probably many persons know the term but can't tell you what the letters stand for.

Just to keep our edge, we make up our own secret passwords now and then. How many of us have not pondered what a colleague meant when she wrote a series of capital letters interspersed with slashes, dashes, or dots? I have my own personal passwords. *I* know what I mean, but I can see myself in court explaining to the jury the significance of "TWW" (toes warm and wiggly).

In addition, there are *signs.* A physician cannot have a successful death unless some physical phenomenon bears his or her name when he or she is gone. Just look up "sign" in a medical dictionary. The number is staggering. Of course, we emergency care providers have a few signs not listed in Taber's or Dorland's dictionary. The positive Samsonite sign comes to mind: the patient who brings a suitcase is planning to stay; the length of stay is multiplied logarithmically by the number of suitcases, as is the determination to stay.

Residents are good for signs. It's a matter of pride to be able to recite as many signs as possible in their patient assessment litanies. Next time you are involved in a patient discussion with a resident, throw in a couple of signs all your own. The odds are that they will come back to you a few days later. Signs are good passwords when you are trying to gain official membership into the club.

Not to be outdone, some of our patients have developed a secret language all their own. It takes just a little while to know the true meaning of, "I'll level with ya, nursie; I had a 'couple' drinks tonight." And there is a well-traveled, really *bad* guy named "Somedude," as in, "Who shot you? "Somedude." We quickly learn that the date given for the last menstrual period does not relate to the calendar as we know it. And the estimate of blood loss increases at a fantastic rate when it is your own blood being discussed. Finally, we learn to beware of any patients who list more than five drug allergies: they know the health care passwords better than we do.

You just can't belong to the emergency care club unless you know your URIs from your STDs. And remember, if you c/o SOB et CP et HA et loose BMs et LLQ pain et nonprod cough × 6 mo, you are just a LOL in NAD.

---

*Reprinted from Journal of Emergency Nursing, ©1989; 15(4):360 with permission from Mosby-Year Book, Inc.

How to Present a Mortality and Morbidity Conference*

IRVING L. KRON, M.D.

The Mortality and Morbidity Conference is the forum in which the surgical resident presents complications. To avoid excessive humiliation to the resident physician, various ploys have been used to spread the blame for bad results. I have taken the liberty of numbering these in order of frequency of use, as well as following each ploy with an interpretation.

1. Blame it on the anesthesia: This is a very effective means of transferring blame, in that attending surgeons will accept as gospel anything bad said about anesthesiologists.

2. Blame it on the patient: This technique is particularly effective when the patient is an antisocial personality (dirtball). The implication is that, if the patient had followed the physician's orders, the disastrous results would not have occurred; e.g., his leg would not have become infected and required amputation, if he had just stopped chewing tobacco.

3. Blame it on nursing: This is more problematic in a southern university where chivalry is still alive. However, most bad results can be blamed on a "lazy" nurse who did not inform the doctor in time to avoid the complication (even if the complication was unavoidable).

If these straightforward diversions don't seem as if they'll fly, one may have to resort to more complicated efforts to cloud the issues.

4. Focus the discussion on an interesting part of the case that has nothing to do with the complication: e.g., even though the patient was drawn and quartered, the fact that the autopsy showed two spleens could be played up to avoid discussing the obvious complication.

5. Ask one of the attending doctors for his technique for handling the complication. This is a particularly effective technique, although not well known. Present the horrendous complication and then ask the most arrogant attending in the room the following: "Dr._____, you have a great deal of experience with this complication. How would you manage it?" Invariably the attending physician will begin to expound on the complication and its management, waxing his most eloquent just prior to realizing he's been had.

6. "It was God's will": i.e., despite maximum attempts, the patient died and is probably better off. This works best at religious-affiliated universities.

7. "Dazzle them with curve balls." When you have a particularly bad complication, first present several minor and possibly even nonexistent complications in great detail, hoping the audience will become so bored they won't catch the real complication.

8. Discuss unrelated physiology: e.g., after you have severed the patient's aorta, causing his rapid demise, discuss the death as due to a low serum iron level. This works best if you bring in multiple irrelevant and occasionally fabricated references in the literature, allegedly supporting your viewpoint.

9. Explain that you gave the patient and family informed-consent warning about the risks of the procedure. However, this is a particularly nervy (read: questionable) technique wherein one attempts to sidestep the complication by implying that warning the patient of the risks absolves one of all guilt.

10. Throw yourself on the mercy of your colleagues. If there is no way out, beg forgiveness. This is a surprisingly effective technique, although rarely used.

N.B.: There is only one excuse that can never be used in academic circles. *Never* blame the attending surgeon, no matter how much he is at fault.

*Reprinted from Journal of Irreproducible Results, ©1985; 30(3):5. Reprinted by permission of Blackwell Scientific Publications, Inc.

How Well Do You Communicate?*

MANCHESTER RADICAL NURSES GROUP

Nurses and Patients

A patient tentatively asks, "Am I dying, nurse?"
Do you say:
(a) "You'll feel better after a bath."
(b) "We all have to go sometime, Mr. Smith."
(c) "Of course not."
(d) "Yes"

A patient asks, "What are these white tablets for, nurse?" Do you say:
(a) "To make you feel better, Mrs. Thomas."
(b) "To change the way your hormones work."
(c) "It's diethylstilboestrol, Mrs. Thomas."
(d) "I don't know, I've never heard of them."

A patient asks, "How will I feel after the operation, nurse?" Do you say:
(a) "Try not to think about it."
(b) "You'll feel much better after a bath."
(c) "You'll have to ask the doctor."
(d) "You'll only have one or two tubes."

A patient says, "I'm feeling tense nurse!"
Do you say:
(a) "I'll get the doctor to change your medication."
(b) "You'll feel much better after a bath."
(c) "Would you like to see the chaplain?"
(d) "*You're* feeling tense?!"

A patient calls, "Nurse, I think I'm bleeding!"
Do you say:
(a) "Mention it to the doctor on her next round."
(b) "Not just now, Mrs. Jones."
(c) "You'll feel much better after a bath."
(d) "Well are you or aren't you?"

Nurses and Doctors

A consultant asks you to make him a cup of coffee.
Do you say:
(a) "I'd love to."

(b) "As a doctor I'm surprised you don't know that an excessive intake of caffeine is harmful and I'm not willing, at the moment, to participate in your destruction."
(c) "The patients have just had breakfast and if there's any tea left in their pot you can help yourself."
(d) "I am here to look after the patients and not to pander to your every little whim!"

A consultant insists on shouting at the patients during her ward round. Do you:
(a) Join in and shout with her.
(b) Ask the patients if they heard the doctor all right.
(c) Ask how long she's had her hearing problem.
(d) Shout back at her when you have something to say.

A doctor continually calls you "My dear" each time he comes onto the ward. Do you:
(a) Say, "Isn't it nice we have such a good work relationship?"
(b) Mutter ancient curses under your breath.
(c) Say, "Yes I can see working with me must cost you a lot."
(d) Say, "Yes, my dove?"

You're teaching a first year nurse how to do a particularly difficult dressing when a doctor tells you he wants you to chaperone him immediately. Do you say:
(a) "Yes of course," drop everything and run?
(b) "I'll be finished in about an hour and a half."
(c) "Will you book an appointment with the ward clerk?"
(d) "What, have you offended *ALL* the other nurses?"

A patient is bleeding heavily from his operation site. You've informed the doctor but she's taking no notice. Do you:
(a) Say, "Perhaps it is nothing to worry about."
(b) Disclaim responsibility for the patient's future welfare.
(c) Threaten to get in touch with the senior registrar.
(d) Get in touch with the senior registrar.

*Reprinted from Nursing Times, ©1983; 79(51):62–63 with permission from Macmillan Magazines, Ltd.

Nurse to Nurse

It's your first day on a new ward having just left a geriatric ward and you ask Sister to explain about each patient. She says there isn't time. Do you say:
(a) "Sorry to trouble you."
(b) "Well then I'd like to look at the Kardex."
(c) "Well, I suppose there's not much difference between geriatrics and surgery, is there?"
(d) "Oh, are we too busy to work with the patients today?"

You've just been asked to do a procedure you've never done before. Do you:
(a) Say nothing and hope you get it right.
(b) Grab the procedure book and hide in the sluice.
(c) Say, "I know it's silly but I can't remember how to do this."
(d) Say you refuse to do any procedure for which you haven't had adequate instruction.

A nursing officer comes onto the ward and says she's had complaints about your attitude to doctors. Do you:
(a) Apologize profusely.
(b) Demand to know which doctors have complained.
(c) Deny all knowledge of ever having spoken to a doctor.
(d) Dare her to tell the doctors to see you themselves.

A new student has just come onto the ward and you know she's feeling unconfident. Do you:
(a) Say, "We all have to go through it" and leave her to it.
(b) Say, "Come on, cheer up."
(c) Say, "Don't worry, it gets better after the first two years."
(d) Work with her all day and suggest she comes with you to the Radical Nurses' meeting that evening.

A male student nurse tells you he's discriminated against in nursing. Do you say:
(a) "Yes, it must be very hard for you boys."
(b) "I don't mind you doing my share of the bed baths if you feel you're being left out."
(c) "Perhaps you could ask for proportional representation in the Rcn?"
(d) "Never mind, I'm sure you'll make up for it when you're a nursing officer in a couple of years time."

How the *Write* Stuff Can Go Wrong*

AVICE H. KERR, R.N., B.A.

Some say the boundary between comedy and tragedy is as fine as a spiderweb. That's especially true of charting, where errors can be funny . . . or fatal.

As you'll see from the following examples (all taken from actual records), charting errors fall into certain patterns. By reading between the lines, perhaps you'll not only get a few chuckles but also discover ways to keep your charting accurate.

Changing Gears

Sometimes nurses seem to let their minds slip into "neutral" when doing routine charting, leading to entries such as these: "dressings dry and intact with moderate serosanguineous drainage"; "back pain in the neck and head"; and "respirations deep and regular—no breath sounds."

* Reprinted with permission from the January issue of Nursing 1987, ©1987; Springhouse Corporation, Springhouse, Pa. 19477. All rights reserved.

Certainly, only momentary inattention (or magic) could have led to this startling report, "Elbow got better, then disappeared."

Professional Mistakes

Attempting to write in a more professional manner can produce very unprofessional results. Plain English *communicates* more than the nursing "buzzwords" that are briefly fashionable, then replaced by new ones. Consider "verbalize."

What does a note such as "Patient is not verbalizing pain" mean? Does the patient have no pain, or is he simply not talking about it? Better to use the clearer (and less pretentious) "Patient says he has no pain."

"Professionalizing" one's writing usually results in awkward constructions, such as "Exquisite care taken when turning"; "When pain is remitted, it is not entirely remitted"; "Patient states slight relief as stated when asked"; "Burn covers back majorly"; "Child denies diplopia." (What child ever *heard* of diplopia?)

Used inappropriately, "professional" language can create other absurdities, as in the case of the male patient with severe abdominal ascites who was described as "buxom."

Or take the word "prone," which means "face down." Some record keepers use it to indicate any flat position; for example, "patient lying prone on back."

Others use Latin words or phrases without understanding their literal meaning. "Admitted per pedis," for instance, has no advantage over "admitted walking"—and it could make those reading the chart suspect the patient was dragged in "by the feet."

The moral: Don't try to be erudite; just try to be right.

Hearing Problems

Because much of the medical record is transcribed from tape recordings, typos crop up frequently—for example, "do to" for "due to," or "graph" for "graft."

Other errors stem from the transcriber's unfamiliarity with medical terms. Typical examples: "transfers" for "transverse"; "fasses" for "feces"; "military tuberculosis" for "miliary tuberculosis"; and "abdominal mess" for "abdominal mass."

But then, transcribers aren't alone in spelling unfamiliar words by sound. A nurse who's heard certain words in a discussion, then tries to approximate what she thinks she's heard, may write "paradoxical" for "paroxysmal"; "epidermal hemorrhage" for "epidural hemorrhage"; and "prostatic" for "prosthetic."

Harder to account for are the misused or misspelled words that any schoolchild should know. A few examples: "quite" for "quiet"; "patient can't here"; "child seen hear last week"; or "mussels" for "muscles."

Despite her idiosyncratic spelling, one nurse's enthusiasm for her patient's improvement is clear in "patient is mutch, mutch better." Frequently, however, misspellings of nonclinical terms in a medical record create unnecessary puzzles in what should be an easily understood communication tool.

Only after several rereadings did the meaning of "arms full of scraps" emerge: The patient had abrasions (scrapes) all over her arms.

Of course, misspellings of clinical terms can have far more serious effects. Think what might have happened if these errors hadn't been caught: "tracheorrhaphy" (suturing the trachea) for "trachelorrhaphy" (suturing of the lacerated cervix uteri), or "hyphemia" (blood deficiency) for "hyphema" (hemorrhage within the eye's anterior chamber).

Letters Im-perfect

When used correctly, abbreviations can decrease the total amount of writing done in a day; used incorrectly, they spark a special brand of charting chaos. For example, the definition of "PERLA" is "pupils equal and react to light and accommodation." But who would know that from the following entries: "PERLA, right eye swollen shut—unable to examine" or "PERLA, pupils dilated and fixed"?

Then there's the matter of interpretation. For example, "B – M + " on a delivery record was interpreted as "baby minus, maternal plus (pH difference)." But any obstetric nurse can tell you it means "baby is Rh negative and mother is Rh positive."

In another example, a typist translated "P's palp," not as "pedals, palpable," but as "petals palpitated." (Guess the patient was in blooming health.)

Many abbreviations, of course, have several legitimate meanings. A nurse who sees "CVA" on a chart and who generally uses it for "cerebrovascular accident" may not realize that in this case it stands for "costovertebral angle."

Follow this rule, then, in using abbreviations: "If in doubt, spell it out."

Wrong Measurements

If patients knew how easily someone could confuse the symbols for dram (3) and ounce (3), or substitute "mg" (milligram) for "mcg" (microgram), they'd be more nervous about being hospitalized. But if they saw how often names of medications are misspelled, they'd be terrified. In one record, Diuril (chlorothiazide) was spelled three different ways on a single page: "Diarel," "Diarell," "Direll." (That's a fairly common drug . . . what about unfamiliar ones?)

Sometimes, the mistakes made involve the timing of the dosages. Suppose a patient (you or I) were given the wrong medication in the wrong dose at the wrong time.

That could be deadly serious.

Other records reveal a disconcerting lack of judgment. After performing surgery on a patient's severely injured hand and arm, the surgeon wrote an order for "neuro checks q 15 min for 2 hours, then contact me." The charting entries showed that, every 15 minutes, the nurses faithfully checked the patient's pupils—*only* his pupils.

In some instances, whether the problem is improper care or incomplete charting is hard to tell. A patient's orders read "Ace wrap to full length of both legs to prevent swelling." His nurse charted, "Ace wrap to feet."

A chart may not tell the whole story in other ways. For example, one entry said, "Patient does not know how long he's been sitting in the chair." A disoriented patient? No. Further investigation revealed that this elderly man was blind and had no radio or other means of keeping track of the passage of time.

Perhaps even more unsettling are the notes that reveal disturbing attitudes: "Patient asks for medicine—even when it isn't time yet." The unspoken message: "How dare he complain of more pain than we think he should be having?"

Picture This

On occasion, the errors unintentionally suggest funny images or reveal hidden truths. A few examples: "Patient struck by a truck on a bicycle" (now that's either a tiny truck or a *big* bike); "Doctor visited—no other problems"; "Patient awakened for medication—not complaining before that."

Of course, sometimes you have to know more of the story to catch the joke. One nurse's slip of the pen, "public area" for "pubic area," brought chuckles when it turned out that the patient was a prostitute.

In another case, an RN wrote that the patient had refused his medication because he was "afraid of addition." That was quite an unusual fear, especially since the patient was a professor of mathematics.

Not Just a Nursing Problem

Nurses, of course, aren't solely responsible for the content of a medical record, nor for its errors. Two entries by doctors, for example, demonstrated that the metric system still mystifies many: An orthopedic surgeon wrote that he had "excised 80 cm, right clavicle," while a neurosurgery resident jotted down this assessment: "right pupil, 5 cm and fixed."

Or consider this patient history, taken by a nursing assistant: "Patient doent have much history—just furnence blow up when he light match."

Surprisingly, poor grammar isn't confined to charts written by those who have the least education or those who speak English as a second language. Even those whose degrees indicate many years spent in school freely interchange nouns and verbs, or adjectives and adverbs. Some examples: "continuous to sleep"; "loosing weight"; "got relieve from medication"; "does not take advise."

Charting Chuckles*

BARBARA WYAND WALKER, R.N., B.S.N.

How would you care for a patient with "pelvic infla-tionary disease"? That's just one of the intriguing conditions I've come across while reviewing charts in my work as an infection-control nurse. The occasional misspelling or misunderstood dictation can certainly brighten routine surveillance for nosocomial infec-tions. Several years ago, I started writing the funnier errors down.

I've now collected so many I can group them. The categories range from the unusual ("He infiltrated the air around the operative site with Xylocaine"), to the unprecedented ("The patient was elevated at the out-patient clinic"), to the unimaginable ("right leg *eter-nally* rotated").

Then there are the confusing on a grand scale: "Serial monitoring of chest x-rays showed hypernatre-mia with normal liver function" and ". . . large, benign chest removed from the pelvis." And the rather surpris-ing: ". . . found to have massive splenomegaly, which was treated with splenomegaly." Some take a reading or two—aloud—to decipher: "At this point, her eyes, nose looked balanced." (Substitute "I's and O's" for "eyes and nose" and it makes sense.)

Admission diagnoses are prime targets for the Error Gremlin. The patient admitted for a "bog bite" was attacked by a German shepherd, not a cranberry. Sim-ilarly, the patient with an "uncontrollable couch" needed an antitussive, not an exorcist. And of course, the woman suffering from "hyperamnesia of pregnancy" was admitted to obstetrics, where presumably she was reminded of her condition.

If we could all only see what some busy nurses claim they've seen. "Fowl smelling urine" makes me picture a chicken sniffing a drainage bag. The patient who "ate half a tray for lunch" *must* have been hungry. Imagine "skeleton traction." Or a patient sleeping on an "egg-shell mattress"—sleeping lightly, I'll bet.

Other interesting scenes include the patient who "looked dusty," the "I.V. found absorbed by RN," and the "patient resting in bed with visitors." My favorite, even though it's gruesome, is "patient seeping quietly." He must have had "serious sanguineous drainage," indeed.

I sometimes wonder, how did they do that? "Bowel sounds in all four lobes." And, likewise, I wonder, why did they do that? "Colostomy opened and CVP inserted."

Although such mistakes can spark some laughs, I think we all realize that accurate charting is important. As nurses become even more careful in their docu-mentation, these errors will become an endangered species—much like the multilegged woman described in one chart as "usually ambulatory and able to take care of all her knees."

---

* Reprinted with permission from the October issue of Nursing 1986, ©1986; Springhouse Corporation, Springhouse, Pa. 19477. All rights reserved.

This Is What the Doctor Dictated*

PETER GOTT, M.D.

Doctors' illegible handwriting is legendary. This can make for poor patient care, when nurses and other professionals are unable to translate medical scrawl into understandable English. With the advent of dictating machines, hospital and office workers rejoiced that this equipment would improve the situation. Has it?

Yes and no. For the most part, transcribed information is legible and useful. However, on occasion, doctors have a tendency to push the wrong button, put their feet in their mouths, speak jargon or use misplaced modifiers. The results vary from amusing to confusing.

The following list, a sampling of what medical transcriptionists have actually heard on their machines, was given to me by a medical-records secretary.

This is what you dicated, doctor.

"Father dies in his 90s of female trouble in his prostate and kidneys."

"Both the patient and the nurse herself reported passing flatus."

"The pelvic examination will be done later on the floor."

"The left leg became numb at times and she walked it off."

"On the second day, the knee was better and on the third day it had completely disappeared."

"A week after operation she spiked a femur."

"At the time of onset of pregnancy the mother was undergoing bronchoscopy."

"Patient left his white blood cells at another hospital."

"Patient was becoming more demented with urinary frequency."

"She had a miscarriage at the age of four months."

"Physician has been following the patient's breast for six years."

"The patient reports that she had considerable pain last night on intercourse in the abdomen."

"She left the hospital nursing her baby and draining clear urine."

"The patient's head was in neutral."

"Husband also relates severe menstrual bleeding the past two periods."

"By the time she was admitted to the hospital, her rapid heart had stopped and she was feeling much better."

"Discharge status: alive but with permission."

"Coming from Detroit, this man has no children."

"Patient stated that if she would lie down, within two or three minutes something would come across her abdomen and knock her up."

"This 14-year-old boy argued with a lawnmower, which then attacked him."

"Patient's abdomen is at war."

"The patient's past medical history has been remarkably insignificant with only a 40-pound weight gain in the past three days."

"This 90-year-old lady was admitted to the hospital as an emergency because of sudden onset of entire left leg."

"Patient is a real gas factory."

"The nursing home where the patient lives was noted to sputter, cough and run a fever."

* Reprinted from Pennsylvania Nurse, ©1989; 44(10):16 with permission from the author.

"The patient is a 71-year-old female who fractured her little finger while beating up a cake."

"Health appearing, decrepit 69-year-old white female, mentally alert but forgetful."

"The patient was sent home in plaster."

"Patient states she was bitten by both legs of a dog."

"Patient was a great white male."

"She was apparently quite active while sitting."

"The patient was seen about four weeks ago by a physician with a urethral drip."

"According to witnesses, the patient was weaving down the street when he suddenly turned into an automobile."

"She slipped on the ice and apparently her legs went in separate directions in early December."

"The patient was admitted to the hospital on the day of admission."

"Patient states table hit her."

"Patient had acute onset of severe Sunday evening."

"Patient has too much sex growth in urine."

"The patient had reportedly been doing very well when, after breakfast, she suddenly lost her right arm and was unable to speak."

"The patient has never been pregnant and denies any reason for this."

"Patient was provoked by the food on her plate."

"Patient was struck by the car in her nose."

"Patient was in her usual state of good health when she felt the toilet in her back."

God bless medical transcriptionists; may their tribe thrive and multiply!

Raw Data*

ROBERT S. HOFFMAN, M.D.

The data consist of dictation fragments collected from hospital transcriptionists.

"Pelvic exam would be a heroic measure in this female, and I would defer this to her gynecologist. He may have special techniques for gaining irretrievable objects."

"The patient is a dwarf and says he drives two-ton semi-truck. I think the patient is lying and he works in a circus. He has unusual tan lines not seen in truck drivers."

"The patient was admitted with abdominal pain from the emergency room."

"This man was brought in by his family because he is getting old and is losing his hearing, his memory and his urine."

"Patient entered for Dupuytren's contracture. On 4/23, her hands were discharged in excellent condition."

"The patient is a 74-year-old white female who was brought to the ER by paramedics acutely short of breath."

"History is somewhat difficult because of the language barrier. The patient has been pregnant quite often."

* Reprinted from Journal of Irreproducible Results, ©1991; 36(3): 25,27. Reprinted by permission of Blackwell Scientific Publications, Inc.

"The bugs that grew out of her urine were cultured in the ER and are not available. I WILL FIND THEM!!!"

"Pelvic examination revealed a boggy uterus ambulating from the cervical canal."

"The patient is a 20-year-old female who presented to the ER after being driven in a car that she had met in a bar and was assaulted by him."

"Patient had her last menstrual period at age 86."

"I will be happy to go into her GI system; she seems ready and anxious."

"He began to drink a great deal during that period." ("One period a word there and the other period a period, period.")

"We have been sitting on this patient for a long time because of his multiple problems."

"She stays at home and lives with her husband and two wives."

"She was instructed to take Valium p.o., q6h until exhausted."

"Physical examination demonstrates a lady who was lying very pleasantly in bed."

"I see no reason attracted to the possibility of granulomatous disease with such a beautiful barium enema and such a lovely terminal ileum."

"Patient name is *Saulosiafolau, Lotiaipuavea*—spell it just like it sounds."

"Rectal exam is deferred because patient is sitting upright."

"Patient was admitted and suffered severe pain by Dr. Girolami."

"This unfortunate 45-year-old woman has known me for about eight years."

"This patient has been under many psychiatrists in the past."

"I have gone over the patient in some detail and I must say that it is a pleasure to see one of these diseases again."

"The operative field appears in good condition with no bleeding and therefore the patient was terminated."

"The patient will need disposition and therefore we will get Dr. Siebel to dispose of him."

"Patient was released to the outpatient department without dressing."

"The patient is to put nothing in her vagina for four weeks."

"The nurse was handed to the pediatrician."

"Patient wears glasses for hearing."

"The patient was somewhat agitated and had to be encouraged to feed and eat herself."

"On the second day, her knee was better and on the third day, it completely disappeared."

The Nunsuch Handbook*

RONALD J. MIHORDIN

1. Remember, you are mentally healthy and your patients are mentally sick. Ask yourself, if you were not healthy, then how could you be a member of the staff? And, if they were not sick, why should they be patients?

2. When in doubt, suspect and expect bizarre or socially unacceptable behavior from patients and, whenever possible, if you must talk to them at all, communicate to them that you are expecting the worst from them.

3. Whenever possible, however, do not tell the patients anything about what you are thinking or feeling. Remember, communication on the psychiatric unit means: They talk about themselves and their problems and you listen. The exception is in giving orders—then you talk and they listen.

4. Keep in mind that being mentally ill means that patients cannot make decisions for themselves so be professional and make decisions for them.

5. Though you may not understand your own thoughts or always be able to make correct decisions in your own life, you are being paid to decide what is best for the patients and tell them what they are thinking or feeling whenever possible.

6. Never say, "I don't know." The patient may get the impression that you are not well-trained. Of course, you may acknowledge lack of information in some medical matters, but the patient does have the right to expect you to understand precisely what he is thinking and feeling and to know the *one* correct thing to say or do at all times.

7. Do not listen to the patient's statements or questions as you would a normal human being. You are expected to perceive things that are not obvious to non-professionals. For example, if a patient says he is ready to leave the hospital and take care of his own affairs, this means he is denying his sickness. Caution is recommended at this point, for should patients make something out of what you say other than what you intended, this is called *neurotic distortion* or *delusional thinking.* Be sure to point it out.

8. Remember, patients, unlike we professionals, do not have ordinary thoughts or feelings. We may feel nervous, sad, or feel like not talking. They have a different set of feelings, like *anxiety states, neurotic depressions,* and *mutism.* Do not use everyday words with patients or other professionals; they may think you less than competent.

9. Patients do not really have the same needs as we professionals, nor do they care about the same things. We care about being rewarded for our positive efforts. We resent being forced to attend meaningless meetings. We care about what, when, and where we are going to eat. We are concerned about how much things cost. We wonder how we can get a certain person to go to bed with us or what we are going to do on the weekend. Patients, on the other hand, only think about these matters when they are defending against or denying a profound, ugly, psychological scar for which we and they must unceasingly search.

10. Do not be deceived by a patient's size, age, life experiences, or accomplishments. Patients are actually little children in disguise. You must forget that they are older and perhaps wiser, or younger and perhaps more sensitive than you. Once they become patients, they become just like children and, once you become a mental health professional, you become their wise, wonderful parent. You may be kind to them, but always remember, as to a child, not as to an adult. Of course, you must expect them to behave as children and sometimes, when they disobey, you must punish them, but only because you care and know what is best.

11. When having a conversation with a patient do not be fooled by how similar it may sound to things you and your friends say or feel. Do not be distracted by normal-appearing behavior. Constantly be on the lookout for signs and symptoms of something pathological that only you and your fellow professionals can see.

12. If, one day, a patient behaves in a way that is unacceptable to others or that he is ashamed of, then on the following day behaves in an acceptable fashion

* Reprinted from Perspectives in Psychiatric Care, ©1974; 12(3):126–128 with permission from Nursecom, Inc. Edited from the original.

of which he can be proud, point out his *emotional instability.* Remind him that we normal people feel and behave the same way every day of our lives. Also, direct all your attention to the problem period, because this is why you are here.

13. Think problems! Whenever possible, focus on, discuss, and express interest in the most difficult, bizarre element of the patient's thoughts, feelings, or behavior. Do not look for normal, non-problem behavior; anyone can do that. Besides, if the patient wants to try to behave in a normal fashion, why should we waste our professional time with him? If he is not crazy-acting, what is he doing here?

14. Professional titles are most important for the staff. Patients have been known to go into severe states of anxiety when they were unable to ascertain whether the nurse to whom they were talking had a B.S. degree or not. Remember, you are a nurse, technician, doctor, social worker, or whatever. Always wear a name tag with your title on it and, if possible, a wallet-sized photocopy of your professional diploma or certificate should be carried and shown whenever the slightest opportunity presents itself.

15. Unlike professionals, names and social achievements are not important for patients. We need only know their diagnosis and their problems. All else is irrelevant. Unless the diagnosis is used and kept well in mind, patients tend to become an assorted conglomeration of individuals, all appearing unique and different. Fortunately, with the aid of the diagnosis, we are able to categorize them and make our work a lot easier.

16. Do not expect patients to speak for themselves. If you are wondering why a patient is behaving in a certain manner, do not ask him. Go to his chart and look for his diagnosis—that will generally explain everything. However, if it does not, you must resist asking the patient to explain his own behavior. Instead, go to his doctor and he will speak for the patient.

17. Finally, expect patients (disguised children) to bring joy and a sense of fulfillment into your life, just as real parents expect of their children. Make them your life. Let them fulfill your needs. If you have a need to be an authority, do not write a book or be a teacher—be an authority to your patients. If you have a need to enforce rules and see that people behave properly, do not be a policeman or a judge—be a policeman or a judge to your patients. If you long for devotion, loyalty, and unquestioning obedience, do not get a dog—get these from your patients.

If you remember these simple precepts, you will be able to walk away from each day of work with a warm, exhilarated feeling, and the joy of knowing that you, a dedicated, sincere, skilled, unselfish, expert professional, have helped in some small way those helpless, hopeless, crazy-acting, miserable creatures we call patients.

Nightingale Records Presents:

Bedpan Blues*

The song collection you've been waiting for!
A dozen of your favorite tunes in new performances
by the hottest all-nurse singing groups.
A must for your next "Recovery Room" party!

You get all of these Great Songs!

Night and Day
by The Circadians

Never My Love
by The Frigidaires

Twilight Time
by The Cataracts

You Make Me Feel Like Dancing
by The Choreatoids

Fascinatin' Rhythm
by The Wenckebachs

The Wayward Wind
by The Flatulents

It's a Heartache
by Ann & Gina

Sugar in the Morning
by The Dipsticks

I've Got You Under My Skin
by The Scabies

It's Not For Me To Say
by The Aphasics

Splish Splash
by The Ascites

and the smash hit
Great Balls of Fire
by Orchitis & The Mumps

This fabulous collection can be yours on LP, cassette or
compact disk, for the incredibly low price of just $12.99

send to:
Nightingale Records
221 1/2 Decubitus Drive
Burnout Beach, Tahiti

Send for BEDPAN BLUES Today!

* By Steven Tiger. Reprinted with permission from Journal of Nursing
Jocularity, ©1992; 2(3):31.

Comments Nurses Could Live Without*

VIRGINIA MOORE DEWEES, R.N.

"I'll bet you really get hardened don't you?"

"Why can't I wear eye makeup to surgery? I'm having my appendix out, not my eyes."

"Are you sure I only get this pill every four hours? I take it whenever I want at home."

"She's one of the good ones, Sarah. This is the one I told you about."

"I'd better behave myself or you'll give me one of those shots."

"I don't know how you stand this kind of work. I'd never be able to do it."

"Have a piece of our homemade salami."

"I've been in this hospital so often I own part of it. I know everybody. What's your name?"

"I'll bet you see some pretty weird people don't you?"

"Why can't I get a beer and pizza before the late late show?"

"My I.V. just ran dry!"

"What kind of surgery did that man across the hall have?"

"I think I'm getting a rash from that shot."

"I know it's three A.M. but my doctor told me I could have a sleeping pill. What do you mean, he didn't write it?"

"Would you like to work a double shift?"

WHERE ARE WE?

Any grade school child will tell you that a nurse means a white cap, a nurse's pin, and sensible white shoes. She is always there with a smile, ready and willing to give you "that" shot.

Since nursing is the quintessential female profession, nurses are often portrayed by the media in the same stereotypical fashion as women. The most vivid imagery that comes to mind is that of angel, physician's handmaiden, sex symbol, and torturer. Thankfully, these deeply ingrained images are not true reflections of the diversity of real-life nursing.

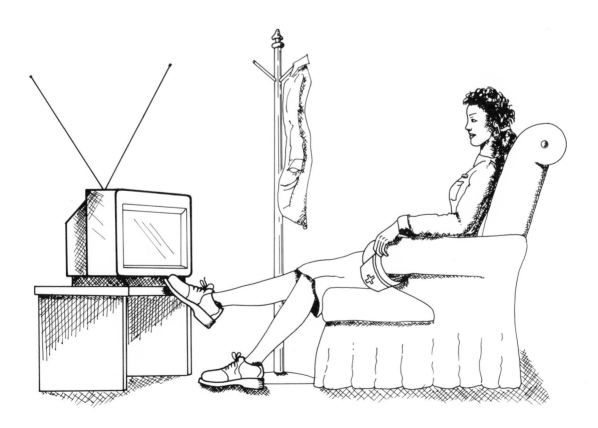

Origins of Nursing Knowledge*

MARY R. INGRAM, R.N., M.S.

In the beginning the All-Knowing planted a garden. In the midst of the garden, She placed the Tree of Knowledge. This tree produced a veritable fruit salad, with many different kinds of fruit growing on each of its branches. There were apples and oranges, kumquats and pears, peaches, bananas and plums and more. And each contained the seeds of a different type of knowledge. To the visitors who wandered into the garden, the All-Knowing said, "You may eat of the fruit of the Tree of Knowledge." The visitors who ate the fruit became known as researchers, and came and went from the garden as they pleased, or as their federal grants allowed.

One day, a visitor strolled to the Tree and inquired about the various fruits growing there. The All-Knowing pointed to a small group of researchers who had just finished eating a shiny, red fruit. "These persons have just sampled the Empirical Apple, a tart, and somewhat dry fruit, which is currently quite abundant. It opens the mind to the wonders of the senses—sight, sound, touch, taste, smell—and induces an overpowering urge to measure the known universe." As the visitor watched, the "Empiricists," as they were called, scurried about with watches, rules and calculators, looking very serious and mumbling a good deal to themselves.

"What is that fruit?" asked the visitor as she pointed to a star-shaped crystal at the tree's summit.

"That," replied the All-Knowing, "is the fruit of Practice Theory. It used to grow on a peripheral branch, but Dickoff and James moved it to the top of the Tree. It looks pretty good there, don't you think?"

The visitor agreed and asked what it tasted like.

"Not many people know," sighed the All-Knowing. "Those who are most interested in Practice Theory are the clinic nurses who come here after working double shifts. They usually manage to climb to the middle branches, then fall asleep."

As She spoke, several nurses in crumpled white uniforms began ascending the Tree. "Let's hope that they get farther than they did last time."

The visitor spied a small group of researchers lying beneath the Tree, crunching loudly on long, woody objects. "Who are they?" she asked.

"Those are the Grounded Theorists. The fruit that they seek is actually a root, or a series of roots, that grow beneath the Tree. The roots synapse with other roots, creating an underground network that spans the entire garden. These researchers spend a lot of time eating roots, partly because they are so hard to digest and partly because of their addictive effect." As the visitor watched, the Grounded Theorists tasted the roots, looked perplexed and asked aloud, "But what's the whole picture?" Then they unearthed more roots and repeated the process.

Another group of researchers wafted by, holding fruits that changed color and shape when passed from one person to another. They spoke in muted voices and empathetic tones and sighed frequently. "What kind of fruit is that?" inquired the visitor.

The All-Knowing smiled. "That is the fruit of Phenomenology. It never appears entirely the same to anyone at any particular time. To one fellow, it is blue and soft; to another, it is green and spiky. Those who eat it become very tolerant of others' opinions, produce copious notes and wander in and out of an existential vacuum for weeks at a time."

Finally, the visitor came upon an exotic-looking fruit with a green skin that looked much greener than any other fruit in the vicinity. "I think I'd like to try this."

"A fine choice," the All-Knowing commented. "That is called the Ethnographer's Delight. You'll find its taste quite unusual."

The visitor gingerly bit into the fruit and was overcome with the urge to finish it elsewhere. "Thanks for

* Reprinted with permission from Image: Journal of Nursing Scholarship, ©1988; 20(4):233.

the tour," she said, munching the fruit and eyeing the horizon.

The All-Knowing watched the visitor scurry away. Dusk was falling on the garden and another day was nearing an end. The Empiricists hurried home to their computers to analyze the data that they had collected. The clinicians in search of Practice Theory descended wearily from the Tree's middle branches, and promised to return on their next day off. The Grounded Theorists were engaged in a tug-of-war with the resident moles over the various roots. The Phenomenologists muttered "But what's the *meaning* of it all?" And the All-Knowing smiled.

Can You See Me?*

MICHAEL A. CARTER, D.N.Sc., R.N., F.A.A.N.

I have discovered the most curious thing; there are times when I become invisible. This happens suddenly, and usually when I'm in an important discussion or when I'm making a patient care decision. The discovery took a bit of getting used to.

Even more curious is that I have discovered that I'm not alone. I've noticed that other nurses undergo this strange alteration, particularly when they offer important suggestions on how to solve a patient care problem. My discovery of spontaneous invisibility has made me think that perhaps the current nursing shortage is really a case of nurses turning invisible. Perhaps there is no shortage of nurses—they just can't be seen. Let me give you an example.

I was busily working with a group of administrators planning for a major expansion of clinical services offered by our family practice, primary care clinic. The other faculty nurse practitioners and I have had some experience at this sort of thing. Our advice was that some of the plans would have to be changed given the demographics of the potential new patients. For example, we argued that the practice should continue to focus on delivering services that we nurses do best and not focus so much on services that would only maximize income. Suddenly, we became invisible. It took us a while to know what had happened because we were still able to see each other. It was soon obvious, however, that no one else saw or heard us.

Now I don't need to tell you how upsetting it is to suddenly discover that you are invisible and don't know how you got that way. I quickly learned, however, that we became visible again when we agreed to do the work and give the credit to someone else.

Having an inquiring mind, I wanted to know if this metaphysical transformation was occurring to other nurses. Sure enough, it's going around. Some nurses claim they are not sure that they ever regain visibility. Some say they notice key times for the onset of spontaneous invisibility. A likely time is a meeting where the discussion is on the relationship of the quantity of nurses to the quality of care. (You can't give quality care if there aren't enough nurses.) Another likely time is when the nurse and the physician don't agree on the best approach to care for the patient.

Having identified the problem, I'd like to present the following treatment recommendations. First, accept that when you become invisible to someone they are not a real person. This may take a while, but remember that real persons have vision and can see the contributions you make. What you thought was a real person is some other life form and doesn't really count very much in the scheme of things. To confirm this point of view, notice how rarely you become invisible to a patient for whom you are caring. They are the real people.

Second, if you suspect that you are becoming invisible, ask a real person, "Can you see me?" Ask several. This treatment is called reality orientation. It allows you to confirm who and what is real and to ignore those things that are not real.

* Reprinted from Journal of Professional Nursing, ©1989; 5(1):3 with permission from W.B. Saunders Co. and the author.

Third, don't despair if all else fails and you become invisible anyway. Keep in mind how much in our lives is attributed to the occult. Use your newfound abilities to create a little havoc just for fun. Nothing becomes so visible as situations that do not go as intended. Use your new haunting presence to bring about change.

Last, always remember, the roadway of life is full of potholes. Spontaneous invisibility is simply one of those potholes for nurses.

"In-Basket" Research: An Education for Educators*

LAUREL ARCHER COPP, Ph.D., R.N., F.A.A.N.

Most nurse educators are invited to participate in research through the in-basket. Couriered from the post office, overnight express, under the door, over the transom, in person or hand-carried from a nephew of the principal investigator, requests come in the form of questionnaires, queries, pilot studies, proposals, projects, prospectuses, surveys, and what might be called propositions. From time to time these unsolicited packets are transferred to one's briefcase—"just in case I get a chance to find a quiet corner in an airport to consider exactly what the writer is asking of me." As an educator, and perhaps as a research educator, one cannot help but see the many "lessons" in these in-basket requests. And through the process a sense of humor helps—on both sides.

The Complex Query. "Attached please find a questionnaire in booklet form. With it is an answer sheet. Please use a #2 pencil only and press firmly. If you are willing to participate please send back the enclosed perforated card. Do not identify yourself. Choose a number. From here on this number will be your own personal code. If you forget your number you may call the 800 telephone number which is listed on the inside of the back cover of your booklet. If you are in a state-supported institution, please omit questions 1–9, beginning at 10 and omitting questions 23, 41, and 49. If you are in a private institution, please omit questions 10–21 and questions 42 and 48. If you are not in an institution, please return this form and ask for

the individual, de-institutionalized, unsponsored query booklet which can be obtained from the following address."

Please Enclose List. "As Administrator/Dean/Director of a large School of Nursing your assistance is critical to the success of our project. We are seeking responses from your faculty members on a project which assesses their attitudes toward their immediate superiors, and we require their names, titles, areas of responsibilities, and home addresses. Please note the stamped, addressed, brown envelope enclosed for your convenience. Please indicate clearly which faculty members are tenured, which retain clinical appointments, and star those who have served on your faculty for more than five years."

The Advocate. "Dear Colleague: This cover letter is to introduce you to my graduate students. Theirs is a most important project. As I know you well you can be assured I would not intrude upon your time were it unworthy. Please read carefully what my students propose. I am sure you will agree that it will contribute to the field immeasurably and to be identified with this endeavor could only enhance your own stature in the profession."

Your Committee or Mine? "To observe the law protecting human subjects, your opening of this envelope indicates your willingness to participate. If your institution has an Institutional Review Board, please submit this request through those channels using the

*Reprinted from Journal of Professional Nursing, ©1986; 2(3):136, 197 with permission from W.B. Saunders Co. and the author.

procedures which have been established by your School of Nursing. If you have a clinical appointment, please submit the attached request to your Medical Center IRB sending three copies of their approval to the three P.I.s whose names appear below. Use the expedited review if at all possible (see the following dates of The Congressional Record.)"

The Student. "I am a student who is interested in doing a study on why statistics should be in the curriculum of our school. Please put your opinion on the enclosed postcard and return it to me." (No return postcard).

The Faculty Member. "We, the undersigned, have been assigned to rewrite the constitution and bylaws of our nursing faculty organization. Please put the enclosed constitution in the hands of the person who chairs your faculty organization and ask him/her to look it over. If a copy of your organizational chart, bylaws, tenure regulations, faculty manual, student handbook and orientation plan is available please send it." (No postage enclosed.)

The Consulting Firm. "The Immediate Feedback Firm has selected you as a leader in your field to provide for them information which will, in fact, provide data to the Shakers and Movers of the Future. Our old established firm monitors the pulse of nursing, but it is only through your participation that policy makers will be enabled to shape our legislative future. As an original source please expect a telephone call between the hours and dates listed below. During this time your opinion will be sought. This telephone interview should take no more than 45 minutes. We are sorry we cannot divulge the name of our firm at this time, but when our study is published in the future we will provide you with a full copy of the text which includes your remarks. If you receive direct inquiries not coming through our firm, we would appreciate it very much if you would share them with us. Post office box number is included."

Dear Busy Person. "We realize your time is limited and we will state as succinctly as possible the ways in which your participation will facilitate our research. Please note that the average time for completing part I as estimated by your fellow faculty members (all of whom participated in our study) is 11.5 minutes; part II will take approximately 29.9 minutes; and part III, the open-ended section, may be tailored by you to fit your schedule."

To The Under-studied. "A review of the literature shows that Deans of Schools of Nursing are an untapped resource and we depend upon you to assist us in the study of Deans of Programs of Nursing. Please help us to understand your motivation to become a dean, your principal role model, your longevity in office, if you had a mentor or significant-other, and what advice you might give future generations of deans. If for some reason the name, title, or address of this questionnaire is outdated, please provide us with the date and reason your predecessor left office."

The Coper. "Yours is a heavy burden of responsibility. Burnout, stress, depression, alcoholism, and paranoia are understandable concomitants to such an office. If you would be willing to share with us your coping mechanisms we are sure that it will enable future faculty members to avoid these pitfalls and your suggestions will be incorporated for others interested in taking similar career paths."

We Promised Feedback. "As you may recall, in 1981 you were good enough to assist me in the study of trends in nursing. Attached please find an abstract of my study. Unfortunately it was never published, but in good faith I promised you feedback. Receipt of this abstract discharges my responsibility as an investigator. I hope you will determine the finding to be of interest to you."

Questionnaire on Questionnaires. Most refreshing of all were the researchers (fellow educators) who put forth a questionnaire on questionnaires. They handed it to me and collected it. Though arresting, it did not contribute to the tyranny of the in-basket! And after all, I am the individual in the airport who watches the professional opinion-taker. Calculating her "random sampling" I go through the turnstile many times—not to glory in my own quotes, but because I am a compulsive student of the tools and methodology employed.

Invasion of the Busybodies*

ANGELA PLUME

Speaking as an essentially practical nurse, I find the endless discussions about nursing research impossible to bear in silence. Now research is a very good thing in its place; there can be few of us alive today who have not benefited from the vision and determination of the great men of medical science. Where would we be without Lister's antiseptics, Simpson's anesthesia, or Andrew's Liver Salts?

But research is emphatically, and undeniably, the rightful domain of the doctor, as the sluice is the appropriate area for the student nurse. Those who argue for nursing research are the same quasi-intellectuals who seek to turn this great profession of ours into a mere technical specialism. You will hear them claiming to be establishing an independent body of knowledge unique to nursing. This is arrant enough poppycock on its own, but it conceals a far more sinister purpose. Their real aim is to make the simple Art of Nursing incomprehensible to its own most experienced practitioners.

Such is the insidious growth in the research faction that we can no longer open the *Nursing Times* without coming across some impenetrable treatise devoted to abstract and totally irrelevant topics, peppered with American jargon and complex diagrams. Fortunately, most nurses are far too sensible to waste their time wading through all this rubbish. They instinctively mistrust research because it so often seeks to undercut and discredit methods which have been accepted for over a century.

Only last month I had the misfortune to have a "research nurse" billeted on me. I consider this an unforgiveable invasion of privacy. This woman, who has scarce been qualified for three years (I made it my business to determine this at an early stage), claimed to be investigating the efficiency and management approach of my ward. This apparently entailed trailing around after me, asking a lot of stupid questions. If she had really been interested in ward efficiency, she could have rolled up her sleeves and got stuck into a few bedbaths. But of course, if she was interested in real nursing, she would never have signed up with the research brigade in the first place.

Frankly, if she had been one of my staff nurses, she wouldn't have lasted very long. No activity seemed safe from her busybodying. I might be carrying out a drug round, and suddenly she would appear behind me like an unquiet spirit, asking things like, "Why is Mr. Reynolds still on penicillin?" Now, as every good nurse knows, patients' analgesia is a matter for the doctors. I am here to dispense medications in line with their instructions; I can hardly be expected to know all the whys and wherefores of intricate treatments, which change from day to day anyhow. Needless to say, I sent her away with a flea in her ear, and she left me to carry out my drug round in peace.

Worse was to come, however. Having failed in her attempts to intimidate me with her interrogation, she turned her attention to the learner nurses. I discovered her attempting to hold subversive meetings with my students in the clinical room. When I intervened she was already passing out "reading materials" which advanced the heresy that pressure area care may be undertaken without recourse to oxygen or egg-white. All the good work I had done with my young girls was undone in a minute. These impressionable young nurses needed much reassurance and coercion before they would return to my tried and trusted methods.

But as I closed one avenue for troublemaking, so she would open up on another front. Her next target was the patient himself, lying ill in bed. Returning from midweek leave, I discovered that she had circulated a series of questionnaires among the sick, which invited them to comment on various aspects of their care and treatment, and award marks from one to five. Needless to say, the mob of malcontents and malingerers who currently infest my ward enjoyed making impertinent criticisms. Obviously those who are ill can hardly be

*Reprinted from Nursing Times, ©1987; 83(47):24 with permission from Macmillan Magazines, Ltd.

expected to advance objective opinions. I want to know when I will be given a questionnaire to complete detailing the frailties of my patients!

The march of progress as personified by those occupied in research must be resisted at all costs. For those of us who do take a pride in tradition, there are some comforting aspects to the research question. With all the research work undertaken, all the forests sacrificed to produce questionnaires, all the hot air

expended in fatuous specialist symposia, instinctive, basic nursing practice has not changed one iota. We are made of sterner stuff.

Every day I leave my ward, 28 patients are the better for it. If the thousands of nonsensical research programs were cancelled, we could afford to pay for more real nurses like me, who care for real patients. The time has come to flush out the parasites: *The welfare of our patients is at stake!*

Nurses: Playgirls on the Boob Tube?*

LEAH L. CURTIN, R.N.

The year was 1983, and it was impossible to find an October issue of *Playboy* magazine. Why? Because it featured a 10-page display on "Women in Nursing." Naturally, hardly anyone read the few words which surrounded the pictures. The article actually wasn't bad: it spoke of nurses' new responsibilities and higher education, of nurses' struggles and ambitions and varied roles.

I first became aware of this outrage when, following my verbal rendition of the American Academy of Nursing's Public Relations Committee report, Anne Zimmerman asked, "Mrs. Curtin, what are *you* going to do about *Playboy?* Another distinguished nurse said, "I've never been so shocked! No nurses I know look like the women portrayed in those photographs!" Feeling was running high, and nurses bought *Playboy* magazines by the carload, and wrote letters to its editors by the bushel. The gist of these letters was that nurses are hard working and devoted to their jobs. We wear flat shoes and starched pinafores over our flat chests. Certainly nurses are devoid of any of those attributes so brazenly portrayed in *Playboy*. "Visit your local hospital," we challenged them "and you will not find one nurse who bears any resemblance whatsoever to those nurses in *Playboy*."

Nurses don't waste their spare time cavorting about boat docks and night clubs. They attend educational programs on their days off and spend their evenings

reading nursing journals. Why, I know hundreds of nurses who have turned down dinner dates because they'd rather study blood gases at home than sit around a candlelit restaurant holding hands with some attractive man. When a woman goes into nursing, she takes a vow of chastity, and promises to devote all her waking hours to carry out the nursing process. Nurses are a breed apart—selflessly dedicated and loyal to their employing agencies. They would as soon think of failing to complete a nursing care plan as of posing in the buff for *Playboy*. Sooner, in fact. *Playboy's* outrageous exposé only played into the hands of those sexploiters who use nurses to profit the medical-industrial complex.

So the argumentation went and so it still goes.

The Nurse as Sex Object

Ever since a couple of sociological studies showed that the entertainment media portrays nurses as sex objects, nursing's "image problem" has focused almost exclusively on the sexploitation of the profession. Nurses' indignation is almost knee-jerk predictable: "We are *not* sex objects" we proclaim. To a certain extent, this concern, while overstated, is valid. However, it seems to me that just about everyone in the entertainment media is a sex object . . . And this state of affairs isn't anything

*Reprinted from Nursing Management, ©1990; 21(5):7–8 with permission from S-N Publications, Inc. Edited from the original.

new either. I can remember rushing back to the dormitory during my student years to watch *Ben Casey, MD*—and it wasn't because he was a doctor. As I matured, *Marcus Welby* started looking pretty good (even though his "nurse," Carmen, *was* a bit of a twit), and nowadays even George Burns gives my heart a little flutter. In all honesty, can any of you claim that the officers on *Miami Vice* have no sex appeal? And what about those lawyers on *L.A. Law*? If they're all "sex objects" too, why should nurses complain? Nonetheless, there *is* a different, demoralizing quality about how nurses are portrayed . . .

The Nurse as Utter Incompetent

It wasn't until I had an afternoon appointment with an orthopedic surgeon that I was able to identify the difference. This is what happened.

My physician, having studied Medical Economics 101, routinely schedules about 55 patients every 15 minutes. Not surprisingly, patients usually have a long wait during which they watch the waiting room television set thoughtfully purchased to distract them from their discomforts. Ordinarily, patients negotiate among themselves to determine which program they want to watch. Our group of patients voted—and I lost 54 to 1, so we watched *General Hospital.*

The scene opened in a patient's room. The patient was a handsome young man about the age of my oldest son (22). He was lying in bed with a sheet stretched over his manly chest and tucked up under his dimpled chin. Although I did my nursely best to do a thorough physical assessment on this young man, I could find nothing wrong with him. The nurse was a—shall we say mature—woman, at least my age. (My fellow patients informed me that her name is Jessie and she's the head nurse.) This nurse was the picture of the "modern" RN: she wore a tailored dress, full-length lab coat with a stethoscope draped gracefully around her neck, and she wore three inch heels.

It was difficult for me to determine *what* Jessie was doing in the patient's room. She did fluff his pillow on several occasions. Otherwise, she minced about the room (in all fairness, one cannot stride purposefully forth in three inch heels, about all one *can* do is mince) and carried on what, in my day, would have been called a "suggestive" conversation.,

In the midst of all this mincing, fluffing and suggesting, the patient went into a cardiac arrest. What do you suppose Jessie did about this patient emergency? Did she do what any self-respecting sex object ought to do . . . i.e., snatch the opportunity for a little mouth-to-mouth? No. She didn't even do what your average American visitor would do . . . i.e., put on the bell and yell for help. Jessie abandoned the patient and minced quickly out of the room, screaming for some character by the name of Dr. Hardy. At this dramatic moment, the episode ended. A brief inquiry elicited the information that Dr. Hardy was the Chief of Staff. Then I knew the kid was doomed—by the time someone found "The Chief," he'd be very dead indeed.

The Nurse as Competent, Compassionate Contributor

Owing to the fact that I'd another hour to wait before I would be seen, I had plenty of time to think about nurses, nursing, *General Hospital* and how Jessie portrayed us. Did it bother me that Jessie clearly had a "thing" for a man young enough to be her son? Was that the problem? Or was the problem that a senior "member" of my profession was portrayed as panicking in the face of a patient emergency, abandoning the patient and screaming for someone else to help? As the mother of three erstwhile boy scouts, let me assure you, the youngest of them would have behaved better. They would have started CPR . . . but a registered nurse runs away?

The real problem isn't that nurses are portrayed as sex objects, but rather that nurses are portrayed as *nothing but* sex objects.

Ben Casey was a sex object, but he also was the best doctor who ever lived. He was doing heart transplants in 1960—on Tuesdays. On Wednesdays he did brain surgery, on Thursdays he delivered babies in the ghetto! He was interested, concerned, competent, compassionate, committed—and making a difference in the world. The cops on *Miami Vice* may be sex objects but they risk their lives to help people, and to make our world a safer, better place to live. The lawyers on *L.A. Law* fight the whole system to defend the rights of the oppressed and correct injustices—and, by the way, they have families and lovers and sex lives which they routinely mishandle.

I have no objection to being a sex object (go ahead America, eat your heart out). I don't mind if people want to think nurses are beautiful and desirable and even sexy. But I do resent it when nurses are portrayed as playgirls on the boob tube: that hurts—and it undermines the credibility of the profession.

Leadership Styles*

JOAN M. WABSCHALL

'Twas the day before JCAH and all through the
  "house,"
The nursing director was fretful and as meek as a
  mouse.
The units were tidy, all ready to share
The kind of leadership that had always been there.
The styles of leaders were unique floor to floor.
There were autocrats and democrats, and then even
  more.
There were "big wigs" and "small wigs," and they all
  seemed to care,
Except for the leader who ruled laissez-faire.

Unit A had an autocrat—a true leader in crisis,
Who was very task-oriented, and had many vices.
'Tho the goal for the floor was formulated with care,
The staff was hostile 'cause they had no input
  there.
Unit B were democrats—as cohesive as one.
They worked well together and got their job done.
They played a role in casting their fate,
With productivity high and satisfaction great.
Unit C was in trouble—there was tension and strain,
For unit C was controlled and led by free-reign.
Though the leader was a resource, she was very
  inactive.
And the morale of the unit was most unattractive.

Yet as the director pondered on leaders galore,
She heard the commission arrive at the door.
They were dressed so decorously; their shoes were
  all spotless.
They seemed all so proper—perhaps even
  thoughtless.
They went straight to work, observing while there
All the subtle little policies and standards of care.

They looked at the climate; they looked at the nurses,
And before they'd leave, the director knew she'd hear
  curses.

> But the floors, how they sparkled!
> The nurses, how cheery!
> The patients, well-cared for!
> The doctors, so weary!

The inspector's brows then knit up with a furl
That made her mind race, tumble, and whirl.
What did he see? Oh, what did he find?
A flaw unconcealed? A mistake of some kind?
"If seems to us things are well within order,
There's nothing out of line; nothing on the border.
But before we depart, there's one thing we must ask—
Just how do your nurses accomplish their task?"

Bewildered, she mumbled, "What do you mean?
The units all function; they're all very clean."
"But what is your model, your manner of action?
Who are your leaders and what's their reaction?"
Then she carefully thought of the styles of leaders:
The autocrats, the democrats, and those
  "in-betweeners."
And she told the commission that regardless of who,
The situation dictated what a good leader would do.

For the unit that shone had not one denomination
But used leadership concepts of all combinations.
And she knew at that time, not one leader was better.
As for each of the leaders, she was glad to have
  met her.
So away to their limos, the commission walked,
And as they departed she heard as they talked—
"That hospital's something, with nurses like that
You can see they know where leadership theory is at."

*Reprinted from Nursing Forum, ©1984; 21(2):91 with permission
  from Nursecom, Inc.

On Milking Sacred Cows*

LEAH L. CURTIN, R.N.

Only a generation ago, expressing an opinion was relatively uncomplicated. The worst one expected was a few disagreements and an occasional comment about one's ancestry. Today one faces not only these hazards but also challenges to one's right to express any opinion at all. Particularly if one attacks an Established Truth, a sacred cow of the first order, one is in danger of being labeled a "self-appointed expert."

To protect myself from such a charge, I tried hard to obtain a post as "expert in residence." I thoroughly scoured the telephone book to find a listing for an Office of Authorized Experts. I looked in libraries and even government directories, to no avail. So, at risk of life, limb and reputation, I sally forth on my own, an inexpert matador, to slay (or at least wound) a few Sacred Cows.

Task Orientation

To begin, I shall attack an Established Truth, *i.e.*, that one must not be "task-oriented." As nearly as I can figure it, being "task-oriented" is akin to being a robot—a professional reactionary, an oppressor of nurses, a dangerous extremist who may upset the conceptual applecart. I know all this, and yet I have an undeniable urge to get things done. I know it's wrong, but I shamelessly admit to a wonderful feeling of satisfaction when I have completed a task. I even make lists of things to be done at the beginning of the day and derive secret pleasure as I check them off.

I am not quite sure precisely how "task-orientation" became the antonym for "people orientation," especially if the tasks are being done to help people. Why should we accept this pronouncement? Who appointed the "anti-task-orientation" people as experts?

One can study and meet and discuss and plan and negotiate and obtain input and bicker for just so long, but sooner or later someone must *act*. To act, one must set goals which must be broken down into objectives which must be converted into tasks. Chores. Things to be done. And each person must do at least some of them or the goals aren't worth the paper they're written on. *No*, the tasks are not more important than the goal. *Yes*, it is most helpful for people to know what the goal is so that they will understand where their tasks fit and why they are important. Otherwise they may not *do* the tasks and they certainly won't be able to set priorities.

One nursing leader (who deserves a lot of credit and whose name I lamentably have forgotten) said, "Today nurses are taught to synthesize and organize, but they can't catheterize." If that's the case, heaven help patients who have distended bladders. Synthesizing and organizing are fine intellectual exercises, but they lose their value if we don't know how to use the knowledge we're synthesizing or if no one will do the tasks we're organizing. Perhaps it would help if we told young nurses (on the sly, of course) that it's okay to be just a *tiny bit* "task-oriented."

Conceptual Frameworks

While I'm in the business of slaying sacred cows, I might as well say a few words about "conceptual frameworks." When I think of the amount of time spent haggling over conceptual frameworks, I get anxiety bumps on my hands. Ordinary folk like me haven't the foggiest notion of what a "conceptual framework" is—which is not surprising because this phrase doesn't mean anything. In fact, the term is a tautology: a concept is an outline of what has been conceived and, therefore, it *is* a framework. Along with other nurses, I am bemused by conceptual frameworks. However, I think that the term is used to indicate a clearly articulated series of relationships among well-defined ideas. Is that perfectly clear?

*Reprinted from Nursing Management, ©1982; 13(9):7–8 with permission from S-N Publications, Inc.

Venting

What is perfectly clear is that nursing has adopted one of psychology's sacred cows—"venting." A form of taking the bull by the horns, "venting" is our new obsession—almost as "in" as burnout.

Loosely defined, venting means blowing off steam—a not necessarily innocuous occupation that could lead to someone's being badly burnt. Sometimes equated with "honestly expressing one's feelings," the "ventor" may blister the feelings of the "ventee." At the very least, uncontrolled venting in the hands of the "let it all hang out" generation leads to unproductive and sometimes intrusive griping. All that hot air could be put to better use driving an engine rather than tooting a whistle.

Although every engine needs a safety valve, its main function is to get something done, not to overwhelm people with noise.

Admittedly, I am a member of the "stuff it all back in" generation, for which there is something to be said. A certain amount of reserve and a degree of modesty in expression can get one through some pretty tight spots. However, I'm willing to compromise. The temperate climate necessary for organizational success probably could be produced by combining the cool airs of the past with the hot air of the present.

Wholism

Speaking of the present, anyone today who is not in favor of wholistic is in trouble. Any nurse who even attempts to put a Band-Aid on a boo-boo will be considered incompetent unless she also finds out about the unfortunate victim's sex life, mental state and socio-economic status. It doesn't matter whether or not this information is necessary for the patient's care or even whether or not anyone uses the information; if you don't worm it out of him, you're not a good nurse.

To complicate matters further, different authors use the term to mean different things—from the Eastern Yin and Yang to the Western touch therapy. Some people spell it with the "w" (wholism), others without the "w" (holism), which leaves one in a rather unholy mess.

I think that the term was originally coined to remind us that patients are human beings, in which case I'm all for it. Certainly patients are not their diseases (the

hepatitis case in 404) or removed organs (the gall bladder in 606) or broken parts (the fractured femur in 203). However, I am instinctively chary of people who think we can crawl inside someone's psyche and turn him inside out during his hospital stay. I'm not sure that it's proper and I'm quite sure that it's indelicate.

Noncompliance

Occasionally, of course, one runs into a patient who simply won't reply to some of our requests for personal data—a *noncompliant patient*. Roughly defined, a noncompliant patient is one who doesn't do what health professionals think he ought to do. Really, it's not surprising that patients ignore our counsel, teachings and questions if we approach them with the attitude embodied in the word "noncompliance." Indeed, why should they comply with what we say if we don't tailor our words to fit *their* goals? We say that we set goals *with* patients rather than *for* patients, yet the literature is replete with articles about patient noncompliance. Now, I ask you, who is failing to comply with what?

Non-Judgmental

Even though we may spend our time trying to figure out ways to make patients comply with a health regimen, you can be sure that whatever approach we develop will be "nonjudgmental." To be orthodox today, one must be nonjudgmental. Perhaps that's part of the problem. Judgment may be defined as "the ability to come to opinions of things; the power to compare ideas and ascertain the relations of terms and propositions; understanding; good sense. . . . " but everyone knows that a good nurse is not judgmental. Somewhere along the line we equated the making of judgments with censure, condemnation or punishment. Yet, *Webster's* dictionary gives the following synonyms for judgment—"discernment, discrimination, penetration, sagacity, decision."

I seriously doubt that I can extract "judgment" from the toils of "condemnation," so I will content myself with saying that being nonjudgmental doesn't mean making no judgments. It means accepting people the way they are, not as we wish they were. If we keep this in mind, we might just throw out the term "patient noncompliance" and start adjusting our approaches to comply with the patient's reality. I think it could work.

Feelings

However, I doubt that we'll reach that point unless we become comfortable with the idea that it's acceptable to *think.* Apparently, thinking has gone out of style. What is in fashion is "feeling." It is quite permissible to feel anything you like—even to the point of spilling your feelings all over unwary bystanders—but if you *think* anything, correct form requires that you keep your thoughts to yourself. It's also much safer that way. No one can challenge what you feel, but anyone can challenge what you think by subjecting it to the rules of logic. Thus, we have administrators who "feel" that the budget must be kept in line, and nurses who "feel" that a patient needs a laxative. I leave it to the reader to determine what or where they felt to arrive at these conclusions.

Unfortunately, I have run out of space before I have run out of sacred cows. A few others that really do deserve attention are "assuming roles" as in pretending (like an actor) to be something: "quality care" for which there is no definition; "human resources" which, I presume, refers to people—hundreds are out in the field. However, this inexpert matador is retiring from the ring, having dealt with enough bull for one day.

I Want To Be a Soap Opera Nurse*

VIRGINIA MOORE DeWEES, R.N.

Some nurses launch careers in intensive care or surgery, but the job par excellence is Soap Opera Nurse.

Soap Opera Nurses never mess around fixing injections, pouring laxatives, or counting narcotics. They just stand there with a minitray of medications and look efficient. They have perfectly fitted uniforms for their size-five figures, caps that never tilt, and stockings that never run.

Soap Opera Nurses invariably date, marry, and divorce doctors, which gives them a headstart in deciphering medical handwriting.

Soap Opera Nurses can always be found in the nurse's station puttering around with reports and telephone messages—seldom in patient's rooms puttering with snarled I.V. tubing or with clogged suction.

Soap Opera Nurses are usually just arriving, just leaving, or just about to take a coffee or lunch break. They rarely write on charts because they're so busy handing them to other people.

When a Soap Opera Nurse wants an elevator, it's always there as are the doctors who lurk near telephones, coffee machines, water coolers, or in wood-paneled offices three steps away.

Soap Opera Nurses spend minimal time with patients but can reel off enough information about them to make a computer blush. They know all the visitors' first names. The only characters who slip by the entire nursing staff unnoticed are criminal types intent on threatening or killing patients.

Soap Opera Nurses never look tired. Their makeup is like the cover of *Glamour.* After work, they whip up a little dinner for six or go out on the town with the chief of staff.

I wish I'd known about Soap Opera Nursing years ago. It's too late now to go back. Besides, state boards are traumatic enough. Competing for an Emmy would certainly do me in.

TV Nurses: Sexy, Deferential—and Phony*

ARLENE ORHON JECH, R.N.

I've been a nurse a long time. Lately I've noticed that nurses on television always look sexy and act deferentially. Frankly, that is not what I learned in nursing school, but perhaps I napped through that part of the instruction. I decided to give it a try.

So I bought a sexy slip, and wore it to work with the lace peeking out the top of my uniform. I copied the sexy, not-a-care-in-the-world saunter that I had seen on television. Then I remembered: I had to count narcotics, take report from the night nurse, assign orderlies, and administer 12 treatments—all in the first half hour.

I didn't want my work to keep me from my true function as a sex symbol, but how could I help it? The phone rang repeatedly, Mrs. Smithers' buzzer signaled her impatience, and I felt frazzled and harried.

In the next hour I administered 45 medications to 15 patients. Two spit them out on the floor, missing my shoes by inches. I could not understand it. Weren't my patients supposed to gaze at me adoringly like the patients I'd seen on TV?

As I supervised baths, stocked supplies, comforted family members, and gave out more meds, thoughts of sexiness faded from my mind. Until Dr. Gillis, the only man other than my patients that I'd seen all morning, arrived on the unit.

He was well into his 60s and hard of hearing, but no matter. Silently, I rehearsed the breathy "Yes, doctor,"

nurses use on TV. When Dr. Gillis boomed, "Where's my patient?" I answered as worshipfully as I could.

"What?" he yelled, cupping his hand over his ear. I found it was hard to sound sexy or deferential while shouting at the top of my lungs. When he still could not find his patient, I wondered, definitely undeferentially, how he found his way to work each day.

At lunch, between bites of sandwich and conversations with families, I promised myself I'd project sexiness in the afternoon. Instead, I found myself holding one patient's head as he vomited, and catheterizing and wiping feces off another.

Hurrying to pass afternoon meds, I paused to bring a cup of soup and a consoling word to an agitated old woman—the first time I'd caught my breath all day. Her grateful smile reminded me that maybe television is all wrong; maybe this is what nursing is really all about. But who had time to think about it? Narcotics had to be counted, charting finished, and report given before the end of the shift.

As I undressed that night, I reflected on the fact that my day had been nothing like the days of the nurses on TV. But I still had my sexy lace slip, and I vowed to try again.

Then I noticed a tiny iodine stain on the lace—and a big red blotch where Mrs. Jones spit out her pureed raspberries. I'll have to watch those TV shows more closely. I must be doing something wrong.

*Published in RN August 1991, Vol. 54(8), p. 104. Copyright ©1991 Medical Economics Publishing, Montvale, N.J. Reprinted by permission.

Nurse Manners'* Guide To Politically Correct Behavior†

ANGELA E. VINCENZI, R.N., Ed.D

Dear Nurse Manners:

I have recently earned a doctorate in nursing and began using my title at the hospital where I work. When I introduce myself as Dr. Flawless, however, the patient assumes I'm a physician and some awkward moments are spent explaining that I'm a doctor who is a nurse. Is there a correct way to introduce myself while minimizing the confusion?

Gentle Reader:

I shall attempt to show you where you went wrong and to propose a modest solution. A major handicap of women in the professions is that they were brought up with one set of manners. A woman is raised to be a lady and a lady never brags, never makes herself conspicuous, never makes a fuss. You are applying social standards to a business situation.

In the professional world, business manners are based on rank or credentials. If you do not use your full title you will be in the position of a woman who has invested in silk underwear. Because it is concealed she derives satisfaction from knowing she has it on and can only share her pleasure with a small circle of intimates. What once was considered lingerie is now outerwear. About this you may properly advertise, not apologize.

But, gentle reader, you assume that clients/patients can tell the difference between a nurse/nurse practitioner/nurse-with-a-doctorate on sight. You may have to explain what a nurse-as-doctor is. And does.

Dear Nurse Manners:

I am a student nurse who is puzzled about the right way to introduce myself in the clinical setting. I prefer to use my first name and my patient's first name because it sounds more friendly but my instructor insists we use last names. What do you advise?

Gentle Reader:

Nurse Manners deplores the current model of instant intimacy with the near universal use of first names. Treating everyone alike effectively erases that which makes us different causing a fatal case of democratus extremus. I cannot imagine Miss Nightingale saying, "Hello, I'm Flo, your nurse for this evening." And her clients responding, "I'm Vicky and this is Albert, we're so worried about our Eddie."

There is no consensus in present-day clinical America regarding names. One person is insulted by using the first name because it implies an unwanted familiarity; another is insulted to be addressed Mr. or Ms. because it's formal. Trying to second-guess the rationale behind everyone's smallest communication has added immeasurably to the stress of modern nursing care. So ask the patient's preference.

Dear Nurse Manners:

I'm the senior class secretary and I'm uncertain about the correct way to address invitations to the reception following our graduation. The unmarried faculty can be addressed as Dr. Perfect or Prof. Awful but the married faculty are giving me a problem (Freudian slip).

Gentle Reader:

The Problem that you wrestle with is how to address a person who was not supposed to exist. You are adapting a European system of etiquette and protocol which was based on court life, where women received the status of their husbands as most wives had little of their own. Further ideological damage was incurred when "Mrs." became properly used only with the husband's name and never the wife's given name. There ceased to be any correct way of addressing a married woman in a professional context.

*With grateful acknowledgement to Judith Martin ("Miss Manners") whose columns and books inspired this piece. See Martin, J. (1982) **Miss Manners' guide to excruciatingly correct behavior.** New York: Atheneum; Martin, J. (1985) **Common Courtesy: In which Miss Manners solves the problem that baffled Mr. Jefferson.** New York: Atheneum.

†Reprinted with permission from Image: Journal of Nursing Scholarship, ©1991; 23(3):193–194.

But we do exist and our excruciatingly correct envelopes are written:

> *Dr. Caring (first name) and Mr. John Smith*
> *Professors Caring and John Smith (both with academic rank)*
> *Drs. Caring and John Smith (each with M.D. or Ph.D.)*
> *Or, failing knowledge of credentials or degrees or marital status: Mary Jones and John Smith.*

You will note I invoked the rule of "Ladies First" which has fallen into disuse in doorway and seating usage. My reasoning was not gender-based but, assuming that most of your faculty are women, status-based. Gentle student, where have you heard that before?

Dear Nurse Manners:

I recently attended a conference at a highly respected university where everyone was addressed as Mr. or Ms., not Dr. Is this a new anti-intellectual movement?

Gentle Reader:

Au contraire! In some scholarly institutions where everyone is assumed to have an advanced degree, the "D" word is not used. It's like having a nose, everyone has one so you don't mention it.

Dear Nurse Manners:

I have noticed that physicians use their title of Doctor everywhere, not just when they practice medicine. They are introduced at parties as Dr. Fixit and when they make dinner reservations it's, "Dr. Fixit and a party of six." My question is: Is it ever correct to introduce an M.D. as Fred (or Fredrika)?

Gentle Reader:

You have stumbled upon another artifact of our European system of protocol. The "good Doctor" kept his status over all cadavers, both the clinical types and the roast turkey dinner types.

Nurse Manners has long held the belief that there is a separation between social and business etiquette. My purpose is not to criticize the medical professions for their obsessive clinical identification; my mission rather is to call attention to the duality of work and leisure that most professionals enjoy. As I am the foremost scholar from the rigorous discipline of health etiquette, I propose the abolition of a class system that believes "M.D." means "medical diety." I remind those affected/ infected/effected that even God rested on the seventh day. The simple idea that everyone needs a personal life should have the highest precedent.

Thus, in normal everyday parlance, an M.D. or Ph.D. is Mr., Ms., Mrs. or simply "Sally" or "Norm." Not being a complete fool, Nurse Manners knows this will not fly.

Dear Nurse Manners:

At St. Elsewhere, the doctors call me by my first name, Hortense. But, I find myself answering them, "Yes, Dr. Hippocrates." Should I insist they call me Ms.?

Gentle Reader:

Nurse Manners fails to see where Ms. Hortense is any improvement.

Nurse Manners is not an old crank and if first names are clearly improving the health of America she will refrain from interpreting every trivial communication as a revelation of moral philosophy. To make order out of the current chaos we must standardize health care etiquette. Clearly, the solution is, "Hortense, did the lab reports come back?" "Yes, Hippo, they're in the chart."

Mother Goose *Nursing* Rhymes by Mother Goose*

GLORIA ROSENTHAL

Jack Sprat could eat no fat,
His wife could eat no lean,
His gallstones and her ulcers
Made them follow this routine.

○   ○   ○   ○

Little Bo Peep has lost her sheep
And can't tell where to find them;
Freud looks askance for it isn't by chance
That folks leave things behind them.

○   ○   ○   ○

Higgledy-Piggledy, my black hen,
She lays eggs for gentlemen;
Gentlemen come every day
To see what my black hen doth lay;
And those who eat without control
Are raising their cholesterol.

There was an old woman who
lived in a shoe;
She had so many children, she didn't
know what to do;
She gave them some broth, grabbed
her coat from its hanger,
And ran out of the house to see
Margaret Sanger.

○   ○   ○   ○

Georgie Porgie, Pudding and Pie
Kissed the girls and made them cry,
That was a crime, you will allow,
The whole darn gang has mono, now.

PATIENTS AND OTHER STRANGERS

Just as the nurse cannot be without a patient, so the patient cannot be without a nurse. They meet as strangers and soon are involved in some of the most intimate of human functions and activities. From these chance encounters laughter often erupts, usually behind closed doors, out of the patient's range of hearing.

This chapter also presents views from the other side of the bed— at last, patients get to tell their story. Patients in all their various permutations make nursing a helping profession. Indeed, nurses are the ones who help them get out on the right side of the bed and leave the unit healthier than when they first entered.

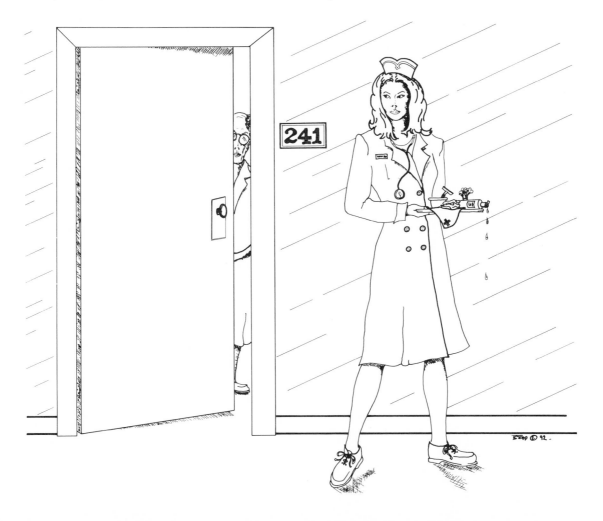

Sex in the Hospital

LEAH L. CURTIN, R.N.

If you think things are bad now, just wait until the State puts a little hustle in your unit hassle. A patients' rights bill to be introduced in the California legislature may do just that. The statute contains a number of provisions, several of which create a legal right to sexual activity in acute care settings. Specifically, hospitals would be required to accommodate all patients' desires to engage in the sexual activity of their choice without respect to marital status, sexual preference, *etcetera* and so on. Those of you who do not live in California (there *is* life East of the Golden Gate) may wonder why I disturb you with a local matter. Ordinarily, I would not, but the opportunity to comment on something so pregnant with possibilities was too much for my self-control—and, who knows, it may catch on nationally.

My imagination positively boggles at the potentialities. Quite aside from the mechanical difficulties (monitors, main-lines, catheters, casts and so forth) and accommodation problems (ordinary hospital beds are *not* conducive to ardor) and irrespective of the scheduling issues (the O.R. schedule can't compare to *this* one in terms of difficulty), there are other considerations.

Infection Control

Just think of its possible impact on infection control. In addition to the more traditional problems associated with the spreading of infection from the outside in, the inside out and, of course, cross contamination, some fascinating not-so-traditional problems may arise. Will sexually transmitted diseases have to be added to the list of nosocomial infections? Could the institution be held liable for, perhaps, a hospital-acquired case of herpes? If so, our duty is clear, and infection control committees must expand their surveillance in many new and interesting directions.

Risk Management

And what about possible pregnancies? eviscerations? cracked vertebrae? Surely risk management will entangle itself in the intricacies of these issues. The text of the consent form—not to mention the provisions of the incident report forms—should make intriguing reading. I am agog at the prospect.

Patient Education

The role of the patient education department also poses promising propositions. Fortunately, resources abound—from Kinsey to Hite—the sex manuals pile high. Patient educators should have no difficulty in recruiting volunteers to select from among competing "How to" books. The decisions that must be made about the attitudes and aptitudes that are desired and desirable—stoic tolerance? epicurean acceptance? hedonistic exploration?—raise serious philosophical questions which require expert mediation. Obviously, Masters and Johnson must enter the acute care arena—and it may be years before adequate data are collected.

Materials Management

Moreover, we also must involve environmental services and materials management. Quite frankly, I'm not sure what equipment may be needed or what environmental controls may be required to provide an appealing setting for the exercise of the multitude of sexual sects: heterosexual, homosexual, bisexual, unisexual, hypersexual, contrasexual, multisexual—all seem to require different accouterments.

When I try to contemplate the eventual involvement of the physical therapy department, my sensory neurons overload. Shall the whirlpool become the hot tub? the exercise mats, play pens? And the potential applications

*Reprinted from Nursing Management, ©1983; 14(6):9–10 with permission from S-N Publications, Inc.

of massage therapy and so on go far beyond the resources of my limited fantasy life.

Quality Assurance

However, the involvements of infection control, risk management, patient education, environmental services and even physical therapy pale into insignificance when compared to that of *quality assurance*. As hospitals are responsible for all services delivered to patients, the issue of quality must be addressed. The conduct of audits (prospective? retrospective? concurrent?) raises enthralling prospects. But, before audits can be conducted, criteria must be developed. Although we can rely to a certain extent on the findings of sexological researchers, the application of their data in acute care settings is—shall we say—inextensive. Clearly, we must develop valid instruments to measure and document patients' perceptions, responses and levels of satisfaction. While I am content to leave the development of the objective instruments in the hands of physiologists and sexologists, the psycho-social education of nurses prepares them for suitable input into the development of the subjective measures. I, for example, humbly propose the adoption of the following rating scale (appropriately weighted by researchers, of course) for measuring subjective response:

Patients, please rate the sexual services received according to the following scale (circle only one).

- libidinous
- luscious
- luminous
- lackluster
- lackadaisical
- lustless
- listless
- lifeless
- ludicrous

The results of such a survey should yield some captivating criteria. I hope that the JCAH will duly note my modest contributions to quality assurance and develop the applicable standards accordingly.

Financial Management

All of which brings us to the bottom line. If hospitals must provide accommodations felicitously furnished to promote optimal atmosphere; relevant health screening of proposed partners; suitable supplies; and requisite education, audit, and quality control measures, some charges must be levied to cover costs. Where these charges will fit into current accounting systems is problematic. I am much inclined to designate such services as ancillary. However, if the services are defined legislatively as "rights," can they really be seen as ancillary? Do they belong in the overhead allowance? Should we charge by the hour or by the procedure? retrospectively or prospectively? Should we seek third-party reimbursement? Or should the services be set up on a for-profit basis?

On one hand, we may be wise to separate such services (at least organizationally) from provider hospital and create a new, profitable subsidiary—the Sex Encounters Department. Appropriately staffed, adequately housed and discreetly promoted, it could become a real money maker. Certainly, the profit potential is well-documented and more or less timeless—even without third-party payment. On the other hand, if the state enacts this statute, patients will have a right to these opportunities, which argues for equal access whether or not the patient can pay. To resolve such problems, an experienced consultant is needed—perhaps the madame from Texas's famous Chicken Ranch will be willing to share essential information about accounting procedures, organizational management, quality control and marketing strategies.

Just where physicians and nurses fit into this schema is not too clear—perhaps to determine medical eligibility (if that's not considered discriminatory), to monitor patient progress (short of voyeurism, one hopes), to document patient response (good grief!), and to intervene for patient safety (hypertensive crises, dislodged tracheostomies, disconnected infusion pumps and the like require immediate intervention—even in *flagrante delicto*).

Enough!

In all honesty, I must say that this entire scenario is more than daunting, it's ridiculous. I am all for patients rights, but enough is enough. Not only is enough enough, it is a surfeit. More than a surfeit, it is too much. Even though I shudder at the thought of being labeled prudish, stodgy or (heaven forbid) non-progressive, I must object. That a hospital should provide opportunity for family—and even "great and good friends"—to reassure, comfort and express affection toward their loved ones, I can see, endorse and urge. That an acute care institution is required to provide a setting for "love in the afternoon" (evening, night or morning), I find a prodigious distortion of purpose and function. Private activities belong in private homes, apartments, motels, even bordellos, but not in public institutions. When a person must reside permanently— or for a long period—in an institution, adjustments should be made for private living in public places. However, there is a time and place for everything—

and an acute care hospital certainly is not the place even when patients have the time. Making sensitive adjustments for unusual situations is warranted, but passing a law that requires hospitals to provide for all people's sexual needs is an unwarranted intrusion on staff and patients alike. If a particular patient feels that he must "sleep warm," I'm perfectly willing to provide an extra blanket and worn tapes of my Frank Sinatra albums—but that's as far as I go. And so, to paraphrase Samuel Pepys, let's put this statute "to bed."

"You Swallowed Your WHAT!"*

JANE THOMPSON DOYLE, R.N., B.S.N.

I was at the desk checking transcriptions when Jonsie, one of our hospital aides, ran toward me in total panic: "Thompson, please! I have to see you in the back room right now." I knew it was an emergency by the fright on her face and the trembling of her hands.

"Jonsie, what's wrong?"

"Tom Vale says he swallowed his thermometer."

Tom Vale, 34 years old, had just had brain surgery to remove a meningioma and was spending time with us to strengthen his left extremities. Unfortunately for all of us, Tom wasn't yet fully recovered mentally.

"Look, Jonsie, I can't imagine anyone swallowing a thermometer. Did you look in his bed, on the floor, on his bedside table?"

"Good grief, yes. There's no sign of it anywhere. I went in and put thermometers in all four patients' mouths. Then, I started taking pulses on the other men so they could get off to breakfast. I didn't even turn my back to Tom, but by the time I reached him, the thermometer was gone. We know he isn't quite right in the head, but he says he swallowed it, and I believe him."

"OK, Jonsie, let's go down to his room and cover all the bases again."

By the time we reached Tom the other three patients had left for the dining room and Tom was lying perfectly relaxed, listening to his radio.

"Hi, Tom. How are you feeling today?"

"I'm pretty good."

"Did you sleep well?"

"Uh huh."

"Jonsie tells me you swallowed your thermometer."

"That's right."

"Tom, are you sure?"

"Of course I'm sure."

"Wasn't it hard to swallow?"

"Nah. It was easy. It just slid right down."

Now, in a general hospital, you usually take brain-injured patients' temperatures rectally. But Tom didn't really fall into this category. Since he was in the rehabilitation unit and gradually regaining his mental faculties, we tried to encourage normal behavior, and we merely reminded him not to bite down on the thermometer. But after questioning Tom, I realized that might have been a mistake.

My next step was to have Jonsie put Tom on a stretcher and move him out into the hall while I went back to his room to double-check for the missing thermometer. Poor Jonsie waited anxiously in the hall, praying that I'd come out with it in my hand.

"Can't find it anywhere," I reported instead. "For now, put Tom back in bed and keep him there until I come back."

I went to the desk and started an incident report. Before I could finish, Jonsie was back.

"My God, Thompson, what are we going to do?"

Tom's X-rays Confirm the Problem

"What we're going to do, Jonsie, is tell the doctor and see what advice he has to offer. But let's not allow this thing to disrupt routine too much. Get on with your other patients and try to calm down. I'll let you know what the doctor says."

It wasn't long before the internist arrived. When I explained what happened and told him I thought the patient really did swallow the thermometer, he said: "You probably ought to increase his rations. It's obvious the poor man isn't getting enough to eat."

"Good night, it isn't funny. If we're right, that man has three straight inches of glass in his gut. What can we do?"

"For starters, before we get all upset, let's get an x-ray of his abdomen, stat. As soon as you get the report from radiology, page me."

Shortly after Tom returned from the x-ray department, they called to confirm that he did have the thermometer in his stomach. I immediately paged the internist. As I waited, my imagination ran wild. I could see the patient undergoing a gastrostomy and could also envision the legal papers in front of me, advising us of the malpractice suit. I felt sorry for Jonsie because it looked as if she, too, might face a mountain of legal troubles, despite her conscientiousness.

Nature Provides a Solution

Finally the internist reappeared with Tom's x-ray in hand.

"Well, for what it's worth, the man was telling us the truth. You can see that thermometer in his stomach and would you believe it, his temperature is 98.6. Yes sir, I checked it myself.

"Tell you what we're going to do. See to it that he eats at least a loaf of bread immediately. Then he's to eat at least four slices with each meal. White bread you understand and no butter. Then, the staff is to go through every stool until he passes that thermometer. I don't want to jump the gun and order a surgical consultation until I'm sure he isn't going to pass that glass."

"Do you really think he'll pass it?" I interrupted. "How can a thermometer safely wind its way through the convolutions of the bowel? Did you ever see it happen before?"

"No," said the doctor, "I never did, but you know nature is wonderful. It may just surprise us and work out its own solution."

Four long days went by. I was at the desk on a Saturday morning when all of a sudden I heard hoots and laughter from the far end of the unit. Before I could get out of my chair Jonsie was upon me. "He passed it. It isn't even broken. Look, Thompson, it still reads 98.6."

Lessons learned: Never underestimate—or fail to guard against—the likelihood that the improbable will happen; never underestimate the body's ability to heal itself; and never underestimate your patients' ability to turn an uneventful shift into a harrowing, yet thoroughly human comedy.

Take a Big Breath, Hold It, And . . . Burst Out Laughing*

JOAN PERRY, R.N.

Not many labor nurses fell into obstetrics by chance because the personnel office had an opening in the labor and delivery unit. As labor nurses now, we probably knew what we wanted to do long before we started nursing school. We are a completely different breed from other nurses. We can stroll through an orthopaedic unit and say, "Thank heavens I don't have to work here." Conversely, a surgical nurse hearing a woman let out a final perineal war whoop in a labor room—absolute music to a tired obstetrician's ears—may not understand how anyone could work amidst such madness.

Although fetal maternal medicine has made great strides in the last ten years, actual labor support is still as much, if not more, of an art than a science. An experienced labor nurse can often tell more about how far along into labor a woman is by spending the first ten minutes talking with her than a doctor can by quickly doing an internal exam. In no other department do we learn to trust our judgment and our senses as much as in L&D. Day after day you can hear trained professionals say, "I have a feeling about this one. She's going to go fast." Certainly this is not a place for practitioners who like to work strictly by the book.

Only in a labor and delivery unit do we get to be an invited guest in a family's emotional peak experience, and then to be thanked. "We couldn't have made it without you," they say. We know they would have, but isn't it lovely to get an immediate reward for the time, worry, back rubs, handholding and emotional wear and tear nurses put into helping a new mother get through labor?

Being a guest at such a physically and emotionally charged time can give some fascinating glimpses into unique personalities. Sometimes the language people use under stress is shocking. I know of one father who pulled a gun on the nurse because she was letting his wife suffer. Couples can fall apart during a long labor, or amaze everyone with their inner strength under duress. But at a time when they are worried, tired, excited, and not completely understanding of everything that is happening, I think most people are just plain funny! They don't plan to be . . . they just are. Some days an L&D nurse would be hard-pressed if she couldn't excuse herself quietly, leave the room, shut the door, and burst out laughing.

At one hospital where I worked, we kept a journal of things that happened. Notes were made of engagements, weddings, births and special achievements. Newspaper articles were pasted in. The best part of the book, though, were the funny things said and done by patients and staff. Everyone could be kept humble knowing that their greatest blunders would be entered anonymously into the *Commun-i-cation Book*. We each had our favorite item, but a few always brought laughs.

April: Phone call from a patient's mother, "My daughter wants to know if she has one boy ovary and one girl ovary."

June: From a new mother who had been transferred from another county because of complications, "Them there doctors back home may be good, but they sure do hide it well."

August: New father to his family, "One minute he was in there and the next minute he came out . . . just like a human being or something."

Smiles to Dr. Hill for dropping his beeper in the commode his first night on call.

*Reprinted from Point of View, ©1988; 25(1):19 with permission from Ethicon, Inc. Edited from the original.

September: Doctor to mother waking up after a C-section, "Congratulations! You have a healthy baby girl!" Mother, still groggy from anesthesia, "I do? Well, what's her name?"

Father to newborn after a normal birth, "Boy, I'm sure glad you came out okay. I was beginning to think you were in the cesarean section."

October: Husband limping out to talk to the nurse, "You're going to have to give her something for pain. She just hit me in the *!*!*!!"

November: New mother in the recovery room after epidural had been redosed, "I feel wonderful! For the first time in months I'm tingling all over."

December: Young father to his family after misunderstanding the explanation of fetal monitoring, "Things have been going kind of slow so far but they should speed up now that they have put on that electronic dilator!!"

Take Time to Laugh*

CATHLEEN HUCKABY, R.N.

"DID YOU HEAR the one about. . . ?"

Perhaps the only sense we nurses truly can't do without in our day-to-day work is a well-developed sense of humor. During my 7 years as a registered nurse, I know mine has helped keep me sane . . . and carried me through some very long shifts. In fact, I'm considering writing a book based on some of my own experiences and the anecdotes I've collected from other nurses throughout the country.

The funniest stories seem to come from patients and their questions. (*Patients* say the darndest things?) Here are a few of my favorites.

Nurses in the emergency department at Woodland Park Hospital in Portland, Oregon, report a series of unusual phone calls:

A worried man asked, "What should I do? My spare rib hurts when I breathe."

Then there was the teen who wondered, "How can I get a cast? I just want to try one."

Another call was from an anxious mom whose 3½-month-old daughter repeatedly stuck her tongue out. The mother wanted to see a "specialist in that area." The nurse handling the call was tempted to admit she couldn't place the specialty—though it was right on the tip of her tongue.

Pity the nurse who had to field this intriguing question: "How long does it take to get over gamma globulin? My girlfriend has it." Or this: "What kind of drink gives you the most electric lights?"

Of course, health care terms, so familiar to us, can easily confuse patients. I once heard an angry psychiatric patient loudly insist: "I am not psychoceramic!"

Marie Randolph, RN, a staff nurse at Howard University Hospital in Washington, D.C., wrote to me about another "jargon" mix-up: An emergency department nurse handed an elderly gentleman who had a gastric ulcer a referral slip for the GI clinic. After glancing at the slip, he returned it to her, protesting, "But I'm not even a veteran."

* Reprinted with permission from the April issue of Nursing 1987, ©1987; Springhouse Corporation, Springhouse, Pa. 19477. All rights reserved. Edited from the original.

Medical Education Upgraded*

G. K. STANTON

In the university's effort to promote continuing excellence in our medical teaching program, the medical director has asked that residents, interns and students use the following rating system to evaluate patients involved in grand rounds . . . Patients with ratings 100 and above are considered superior teaching cases and will be granted hospitalization honorarium for their clinical expertise.

Characteristic or behavior	point value
1. Transferred to another service on day of admission	2
2. Stool found under dressing	
at first post-op dressing change	10
with no BM's recorded	14
3. Chart weighs over 2 lbs	2
4. Patient has seizure or hematemesis while checking out for discharge	4
5. Patient sent to ward by admitting physician with diagnosis pertaining to organ system actually involved	–3
if correct diagnosis	–5
6. Pulls IV out	6
in full restraints–with teeth	15
if edentulous	20
7. Removes foley catheter with bag inflated	
5 ml bag	10
30 ml bag	30
8. Urinates on physician	10
on nurse	8
on orderly	6
on janitor	4
on medical student	2
9. Defecates in doctor's bag	10
10. Past history reads "see old chart"	1

Characteristic or behavior	point value
11. Concentration of Air Wick in patient's room causes conjunctivitis among visiting personnel	4
12. Patient answers all questions asked to any patient on ward	11
13. Drinks from urinal	14
14. Toenails cannot be cut with clippers, chisel or drill	7
15. Semi-formed guaiac positive stool found more than 7½ ft from patients bed	9
each additional foot	1
on wall or window	3
on sidewalk outside room	14
16. Regulates own IV	2
other patient's IV	4
17. Bites bulb off oral thermometer	2
rectal thermometer	4
another patient's rectal thermometer	11
18. Hides in closet on rounds	3
19. Found in bed with another patient	3
each additional patient	3
20. Found with dentures upside down	7
21. Decubitus on occipital protuberance	9
22. Develops chemical tracheitis secondary to aspiration of fly	11

*Reprinted with permission from Journal of Irreproducible Results, ©1981; 27(3):17. Reprinted by permission of Blackwell Scientific Publications, Inc.

Hip Remarks*

ROY B. MOORE

A guy who gets his hip unzipped,
The joint with brand new parts equipped,
Lies on his back whilst it is healing
And contemplates the cheerless ceiling.

So there he lies with legs outspread
Spread-eagled on the fenced-in bed,
Tubes into his body leading,
Some sucking out, the others feeding.

To ease the ache of torture rack,
A nurse must rub his wrinkled back
And take his temp and blood for testing
How many pills he needs for resting.

The days and nights drag slowly on—
Then all at once the splint is gone!
And lo, comes exercise with pulley,
And up from flat to upright, fully!

That first weak step on brand new hip
Revives the hope of homeward trip.

The sweat may seep and muscles tremble
But walking? Yes! It does resemble!

Comes exercise 'neath therapist's clutch
And high knee steps with aid of crutch.
And in between the ambulating,
A board is used for supine skating.

Just how can man stand all this stuff
To bring the new hip up to snuff?

Well, day and night, the tedious hours
Are cheered by visits, cards, and flowers,
The gift of friends, the true concern,
The helpful nurses at each turn,
The faithful wife, the God that's good
Who helps a man do all he should.
All these and skillful orthopod
Have made my walk a promenade.

And now, at home, each day I say,
"A total hip? Hip-Hip! Hooray!"

Who Says Being an ICU Patient Is No Fun?*

WILLIAM J. RYAN, M.D.

This visit to the intensive-care unit was different. Instead of standing at bedside as usual, spouting wisdom about status asthmaticus, I sat on a stretcher frantically trying to draw my next breath from a tank of oxygen. Trying to relish the switch, I looked around me as my breathing began to return.

The room was typically cheerless. Its center was occupied by a huge, circular nursing station complete with flashing lights, clanging bells, and TV screens. Curling ECG strips covered the floor, reminiscent of crepe paper after a party.

But as my stretcher was rolled into one of the two-bed cubicles that lined the ICU's outer walls, I realized the party was just beginning. A crowd had assembled in my honor, and my condition prevented me from trying to escape.

One glance at the formidable nurse in charge and I felt even more passive. Instead of a modern cap, an antique doily was attached to her wavy blue locks—with an old bone hairpin, no less. A dark pince-nez sprouting from the tip of her nose accented the no-nonsense effect. This commandant was flanked by a cadre of six nurses—four bright-eyed students, the largest of whom weighed no more than 90 pounds, and two vacant-eyed veterans who seemed to be waiting for clues to their mission in life.

How nice it would be to have the hot dog concession at this gathering, I was thinking. Then the boss nurse signaled the students, who wheeled my stretcher to bedside, and each grabbed a corner of the sheet beneath me.

"Whoa there!" I hollered, apprehending the purpose of their maneuver. No way could these kids hoist me onto that bed, I thought, because there's a lot of me. "Let me move myself," I offered. But the big dame put the veto on that idea. "Lift, girls!" she ordered.

Certain I was about to plunge into the abyss, I closed my eyes and called for the chaplain. My fall, however, ended abruptly—in the center of the bed. When I looked up again, the two older nurses were standing on either side of me, and their duties became clear. Each put a hand under my shoulders, lifted me off the mattress, and removed my pajama top. Next, they proceeded to the foot of the bed, seized the legs of the pajama bottoms, and gave a vigorous pull. After stuffing my nightclothes and dignity into a paper bag, they returned to the rear row with the students.

With no further formalities, the nurse commandant marched forward, clipboard in hand, and began the interrogation:

Name?

Address?

U.S. citizen?

Single or married?

Do you have dentures?

Do you wear spectacles?

This last struck me as a pretty dippy question, since the only thing I had on at the time was a pair of glasses. Then she compounded the felony by asking, "Your sex?" My credentials being somewhat less than impressive, I sheepishly answered, "Male."

A lot of laughs—but even this party had to end. Forming ranks, the little students filed out behind the big boss, leaving only the two dames who stole my pajamas. They promptly bathed me, hooked me up to a cardiac monitor, started an I.V., and decked me out in a gown. This was a frothy, cotton thing full of fleur-de-lis and rose bouquets.

Having thoroughly concealed my masculinity, the nurses gathered up their gear and made for the exit. In a weak effort to reassert my manhood, I called one of them back and asked, "Where's the men's room?"

"There isn't any."

"That's a dumb way to build a hospital."

"Perhaps, but it doesn't make any difference up here because neither you, nor anyone else, is about to get out of bed."

"I can't use a bedpan."

"You'll learn."

"Well, can you at least arrange for some privacy by pulling the curtain across the front of the cubicle?"

"Nope. Anything you do in this unit we have to watch."

"I suppose that's why it's called the ICU."

"Could be."

"Or maybe it stands for 'I can't urinate.'"

That skirmish lost, I lay back and watched the whole war go down the tube. Water from the jug hanging over my head poured into me intravenously. It was time to learn.

When all the nurses were momentarily preoccupied, I brought out the proper utensil and shifted onto my side. But just at the critical instant, a large, round nurse emerged from behind the curtain dividing my cubicle from the next.

"Did your bowels move today?" she wanted to know.

"Yes," I replied, "Of course."

"Adequately?"

"By all means."

"How many times?"

"I believe it was 29."

She jotted 29 on a clipboard, then—after briefly eclipsing the fluorescent lights—glided away.

In the ICU, things are never so bad that they can't get worse. Along about midafternoon, I awakened from a siesta and found I was getting a roommate. Fine with me. I'm no snob. But this roommate turned out to be a strange lady with only one thought in mind—to yell loud, clear, and continuously that she needed the bedpan.

Two by two, the nurses arrived and repeatedly explained that she didn't need a bedpan because she had a catheter. This placated the woman for short periods. Following one especially stertorous scream from her, when the nurses had just begun their song and dance about catheters, the lady sat bolt upright and declared, "There ain't no catheter where I gotta go, so you girls better get hopping." They did, but not quickly enough.

You could bank on a crisis a day. Often, word of one came blaring from the loudspeakers: "Code 99-ICU. All essential personnel report immediately!" The message didn't unduly disconcert me—I merely said a prayer for the cardiac-arrest victim—except for the time I had a very personal interest in the announcement.

My heart monitor had stopped beeping, yet I still felt perfectly all right. Checking under my nightshirt, I discovered that one of the dozen or so electrodes previously stuck on my chest had come loose. Hardly a helpless old coot, I moistened the pad with saliva and reattached it. The monitor then resumed its merry chirping, but not soon enough to keep "all essential personnel" out of my cell.

The first fellow to enter carried a scaffold plank that he tried valiantly, but vainly, to shove under me. The second in line came barreling at me with a portable ECG machine. And the third rolled up with a box that had sufficient dials, wires, and buttons to launch a satellite. With him was a chap who wielded a pair of mean-looking black flatirons. This entourage was accompanied by a bevy of nurses also bent on pulling me through the crisis.

"No cardiac-arrest patient could feel as good as I do now," I announced to the assembled throng while the ECG was hooked up and the flatirons hovered above me. "Thank you all for your prompt service." I then detailed the mechanical malfunction, and invited everyone—giving special attention to the lad with the flatirons—to depart quickly and quietly. Finding that my monitor was indeed showing normal readings, they did.

Shortly after midnight, I was aroused by a great tumult. Nurses were scurrying madly about, yanking curtains aside, and peering under furniture. Finally, I managed to get the ear of one and inquired, "What's this, a new way of taking the bowel-movement census?"

"No," the nurse hurriedly explained. "We've lost the little man from cubicle 12. Nobody has ever gotten lost in the ICU before. I've got to go now and keep looking for him."

She started out, then suddenly turned toward my lady roommate's bed. She examined the lumps carefully—first by sight—then by touch—and whisked the covers away. Sure enough, there was the missing patient, snuggled up against Mrs. Bedpan.

"What in the world are you doing?" the nurse demanded to know.

"Get lost, lady," he snarled. "I'm trying to get a night's sleep."

At this, the nurse pounced on my lady roommate, who was now wide awake. "Mrs. Bedpan, why in heaven's name didn't you ring your alarm bell when this man snuck in here?"

"Why ring? It's the first time I've been warm since I arrived in this ICU!"

Sleepy or no, her bed warmer was escorted back to cubicle 12 and kept cozy with a restraining strap. My roommate got her bedpan promptly and without argument after that. And peace and tranquillity returned to the happy confines of the ICU.

No Peace in Hospital*

JOAN JARVIS

We all must notice how much patients are disturbed. It starts early and seems to go on forever; in fact, to the poor patient it must seem non-stop.

"Good morning, Mr. Smith. Would you like a cup of tea? Oh, sorry, you're 'nil by mouth,' but today you can have 30 ml of water hourly. Sorry, go back to sleep."

Half an hour later: "Mr. Smith, are you awake? Let's just shake your pillows and put you on your side a bit." The poor man smiles weakly as once again he's roused from his sleep. "Go back to sleep, Mr. Smith; don't forget to move your legs."

Then: "Hallo, Mr. Smith. Sorry to wake you. Can I just do your observations? Won't take a minute. Day staff will be on soon; they'll change your bed and make you comfortable."

"Wake up, Mr. Smith. Just going to give you an injection to help your pain."

"Feeling better, Mr. Smith? Just come to aspirate your Ryle's tube."

"Good morning, Mr. Smith. Let's make your bed and sit you up a bit. Must look after that chest. Did you have a good night?"

Properly planned patient care can cut out unnecessary disturbances, particularly for patients who need sleep.

* Reprinted from Nursing Times, ©1982; 78(31):1317 with permission from Macmillan Magazines, Ltd.

The Other Side of the Sheets*

LES DAWSON

When one is being trundled off to hospital, there is an awful sense of emptiness and the mind is racked by such dreadful thoughts as: "Will I ever come out in one piece?" and "I'll bet the surgeon drinks!"

So it goes on in your head as the ambulance speeds off to God knows where. As I was being hustled into the ambulance by a burly attendant with pronounced acne, a friend of mine shouted, "Don't let them cut you up." That did it; I whined and whinged and wanted to go to the toilet immediately.

Once inside the detergent-reeking building, peculiar types kept coming in and peering at me as if I was a sort of freshly landed pike. One grey man muttered, "By Jove, he's fat. Wouldn't like to come to grips with his liver." A large red nurse told me to undress, and then I was bundled into a pair of starched sheets that lay stiffly on top of an iron horror she called a bed. I was left alone as she pounded off down a corridor.

The heat in my torture closet was stifling. I climbed down from the metal rack and tried to prise open a window in order to gulp in some air. In vain I struggled to raise the glass square but to no avail; it felt as if it was welded to the wooden sash. Between sobs, I commenced to clamber back to the pinnacle of the bed helped by a pair of strong hands underneath my buttocks. The hands belonged to a nice man in a white smock who cheerfully held me supine on the bed while he flourished a razor and a small bristled brush. "Come to shave you, old man," he bellowed. I fingered my chin, smooth as a baby's bum—what could he mean, shave? It was only when my jim jam bottoms started to peel off that I realised just exactly where he was going to remove the hair. I was crimson with embarrassment as the blade skied over my private department and I tried to think of golf.

I must have dozed off because I was rudely shaken to consciousness by the red nurse who thrust a mug of scalding tea at me. Without a word she about turned and vanished in a cloud of Dettol. From then on, events moved more quickly than a kangaroo that's just had a promise. The surgeon who was to probe inside me entered the room, growled something and departed with the threat, "It'll be out tomorrow!" A thin woman pranced in and asked me what I'd like to eat. Frankly the menu was more like a coroner's report, but I ordered the cottage pie and apple charlotte . . . wrong. The cottage pie should have been condemned before the crust went on, and the apple charlotte lay in my gut ready to pounce.

Again I dozed off only to be awakened to ask if I needed a sleeping pill. Then came the visiting hour. The wife and kids and a friend of mine with ill fitting dentures roamed in. The kids ate the grapes the wife had brought and the friend told me about someone who had gone into hospital for a small operation and had never been seen again.

I cried with relief when they trooped out and another nurse curtly informed me that I would not be allowed to eat a crumb until my operation. Hunger, fear and suspicion made me dwell on the possibility of escape. Once I tottered into the "Dayroom" only to find several gaunt men with slack mouths gazing eyeless at *Crossroads* on the chipped television. Back once more in bed I pined for a cigarette or a large gin. Ogling the passing nurses was my only pastime.

The next day dawned, the sky was the color of damp underpants and I couldn't chew the porridge. Then in stalked two superbly built nurses who gave me a blanket bath. Oh, ladies, what a joy for the mere male. I wriggled like a minnow and twisted myself into positions undreamt of in the Kama Sutra. "Wonderful, girls," I crooned as they flushed with uneasiness at my delight.

The rest is history. Injected, plundered and pillaged, they carted off my body to the theatre and that was that.

I salute you all, ladies and gentlemen of the healing profession. Keep up the good work, and if any damsel thinks of home blanket bath services . . . I'm your man.

*Reprinted from Tradimus, ©1986; 7(1):13 with permission from Nursing Standard.

Angels of Mercy*

SANDRA L. WREN, B.A.

I always knew they were called angels of mercy. Now I know why. Having spent a week as a patient in a hospital, I had a chance to observe the demeanor of nurses at close range. It was then that I discovered an amazing fact, and now I've decided it's time to tell the truth: nurses actually *are* angels disguised in human form.

The evidence is overwhelming. Only a "ministering spirit," as Saint Paul calls angels, would do the things that nurses do. After surgery, when patients cannot perform basic body functions without assistance, nurses do things for patients that their own mothers wouldn't do. Not only that, they do them with a smile.

In fact, their smiles were part of my second clue to their true identities: nurses positively *glow*. Anyone who awakes from anesthesia, groggy and hurting all over, only to see the kind face of a nurse bending over him, can attest to this fact. No mere mortal could still smile after spending 12 hours on her feet tending to the sick.

Then there's the supernatural power of these angelic creatures. It is impossible to deceive a nurse. They *know* when someone is sneaking a cigarette or roaming the corridors when they're supposed to be resting. They sniff out boyfriends hidden in restrooms and candy bars stockpiled in purses. But they also know just when the pain is getting to you and suddenly appear, medicine in hand and heavenly smile on face.

That's another tip-off: nurses are constantly appearing and disappearing. The latter must be a little trickier, though. I had a nurse named Agnes who mysteriously disappeared. Soon after, a nurse named Helen magically materialized in her place, just when I needed her.

If you think appearing and disappearing are remarkable, consider this: these angels of mercy can change form, as well. When too many visitors threaten to overwhelm a weak patient, the usually benign countenance of the nurse suddenly grows stern and forbidding, and the sweet, melodious voice deepens: "Visiting hours are over for you guys. OUT! OUT!"

Supernatural strength is another sign of angelhood. I saw one petite angel of mercy, a 90-pounder, propelling a burly, 250-pound man down the corridor obviously against his will. He fought all the way, but guess who won? Those angels balance huge loads in their arms and make beds go up and down with a touch of the finger.

Above all, though, nurses have a healing touch. One of these angelic creatures helped me get to sleep each night by rubbing my back with a sweet-smelling lotion. Another infused me with encouragement with frequent, loving pats.

My last piece of evidence may seem trivial, but I think it's worth mentioning. Nurses *rustle*. If you listen very carefully after lights are out and the hospital is quiet, you can hear them rustling as they walk up and down the hallways checking on their patients. It must be their wings, neatly folded under their uniforms, that make that comforting sound.

Only God knows from which part of heaven nurses are recruited. Surely there must be more glamorous jobs for angels, such as making important announcements, like "Peace on Earth!" Surely there are more exciting jobs, such as waging war on wicked spirits. Surely there are more creative, less tedious jobs, such as helping to create a brand new star.

But thank God that there are some angels who sign up to be nurses. Or is it the other way around?

*Copyright ©1988 The American Journal of Nursing Company. Reprinted from American Journal of Nursing, May 1988, Vol. 88, no. 5, page 780. Used with permission. All rights reserved.

REALITY 101

Advanced practicum course providing nurses with an opportunity to explore the role in specialized health care settings. Focuses on the relationship of people/environment interaction, explores wellness, health, and illness as expressions of life processes. Addresses selected problems of the present and the challenges of the future.

Assignment of nurses (by hospital) to day, evening, night shifts, weekends, and clinical areas vary. Nurses receive wages as determined by the hospitals. Continuous enrollment required until termination of services.

Prerequisite: Permission of administrator required. No credits,
fall, winter, spring, and summer terms, all departments.

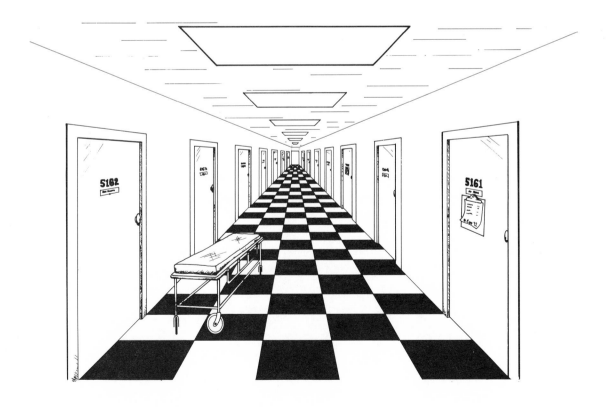

How to
Assess Your Unit
Before You Take Report*

NANCY ARMSTRONG

How do you find out what has been going on in your unit? For many nurses it's through the change-of-shift report, which usually begins with some informal banter:

On-coming nurse: "How bad is it?"

Off-going nurse: "Not bad at all" . . . *or* . . . "Not *that* bad" . . . *or* . . . "This shift will take its place among history's worst disasters—I'd say somewhere between the attack on Pearl Harbor and the Alaskan oil spill."

But finding out about your unit in this way is too short a notice. To get around that problem, try interpreting the clues you find *on the way* to shift report.

What are some of these clues? Well, you can bet your unit is not functioning smoothly if, in the elevator on the way to your floor, you hear the following:

a) Three city police officers ask for directions to your unit.

b) An O.R. tech announces that your unit just broke the record for the number of cases scheduled in a single eight-hour shift.

Then, as you walk down the hall, more clues emerge:

a) Emergency department gurneys block your way.

b) The crash cart is not in its usual storage nook.

c) A float nurse stalks past you muttering, "I'll *never* work here again!"

d) The housekeeping staff is scrubbing a large section of the floor.

And as you enter the nurses' station:

a) No one is there.

b) Too many people are there.

c) Just enough people are there—but three of them are wearing scrubs instead of whites.

d) The unit clerk is there but hidden behind a stack of charts.

e) Two nurses are filling out incident reports.

f) Your head nurse is shouting, "Who wants overtime?"

Now, having interpreted these "subtle" clues, you're both forewarned and forearmed—with a cool head, a calm disposition, and a rational set of coping mechanisms. Besides, how long can eight years, uh, eight hours last?

Job Description
for Nursing Supervisor*

The Unwritten Realities

JUDITH K. PARKER

At Work:

The supervisor must arrive for her shift prepared for any and all occurrences. She will receive a report about the patients' conditions from the preceding shift supervisor. Somehow she must convey the knowledge that she already knows everything there is to know about each and every patient, even though she has just returned from a month's vacation in Florida. The off-going supervisor will be amazed by this ingenious intuition and intelligence.

The supervisor must be the "keeper of the keys," for she must be able, at a moment's notice, to open the office doors, the surgery suite, the elevator, the kitchen, the pharmacy, the safe, the desk drawers, the conference room, the lab, respiratory care, the purchasing department, central supply and, God knows, the morgue!

The supervisor must be ever attuned to any and all emergencies. When an emergency is sounded over the PA system, the supervisor must be able, in a single bound, to leap four flights of stairs and appear on the scene holding her breath so as not to appear dyspneic in front of the staff. Calm, cool, collected, and easy-breathing is the name of the game.

The supervisor must diplomatically convince her staff that they are happy to be working short handed, and then convince the patients that it isn't because of poor staffing that their baths weren't given until 3 p.m.; rather a mistake was made by having too many nurses go on a coffee break at the same time.

The nursing supervisor must know how delicately to extract false teeth from a smoldering incinerator.

She must be able to talk to a comatose patient imitating the voice of a loved one. She must tastefully convince a young man who is urinating off the balcony that the ecologists of the world will be unhappy with his deed. She must be able to delve through contaminated linen to uncover an heirloom lost by a patient.

The supervisor must never show a weakness, such as wearing a lead apron while x-rays are being shot. After all, a supervisor cannot be rendered sterile or barren by a mere machine! The supervisor must show no alarm when a disoriented patient is talking about his visitor who is only 12 inches high; rather the supervisor mentions a friend of hers who is only 10 inches high. A rousing discussion will ensue.

A supervisor never says, "I don't know," when a question is asked. The supervisor says one of three things: "I'm too busy now, but I'll get back to you later," or "I'm going to have diarrhea," or "I'm on my way to the morgue." Then she swiftly retreats to her office and tries to find the answer in Beeson McDermott, Tabers dictionary, or if all else fails, the head nurse-supervisor meeting minutes. Later, when she sees the person who asked the question, the supervisor nonchalantly says, ". . . by the way, about the question you asked . . ."

No task should be too small for the supervisor. She should be willing to start I.V.s, put down N.G. tubes, take temperatures, mop the floors, wash instruments, pick up beer cans from the lawn, tape windows in a wind storm, put toilet paper in the john, water the plants, feed stray cats, and wipe the flies away from the light fixtures.

*Reprinted with permission from Nursing Management (formerly Supervisor Nurse), ©1978; 9(5):37. Edited from the original.

On Games People Play in Hospitals*

THELMA M. LANKFORD, R.N.

Many of nursing management's problems could be reduced if nurses recognized some of the game-playing that goes on in hospitals every day. The games we play include *Hide the Problem, Let's Pretend You Have Power, Who is the Boss?,* and *Kick the Ego.* I am sure there are many more, but these few examples will suffice.

Hide the Problem

In this game, we *know* we have a problem, but we pretend that the problem does not exist because written policy says that it is not *supposed* to exist. To play this game, *all* the players must pretend that written policy is, in fact, being carried out. Example: Written policy states that all personnel must wash their hands well at the beginning of the shift, before and after each patient contact, after using the toilet, and any other time that they think their hands may be contaminated. However, no provisions (*e.g.,* paper towels and liquid soap) have been made for handwashing in patient rooms. Thus, if the policy is to be followed, all personnel must return to the nurse's station to wash their hands after patient contact. This is so awkward and time consuming that handwashing before and after patient contact is virtually ignored. However, nursing administration pretends to believe that such handwashing takes place, and other employees also pretend to themselves and others that they are adhering to this policy.

Pretend You Have Power

In this game, head nurses and supervisors have a certain amount of power as well as accountability *on paper.* In fact, however, power and autonomy rest only at the top of the administrative ladder—but *accountability* is spread out among the head nurses and supervisors. To maintain the expectations of accountability, we pretend that these people have power. However, it is only a myth.

All decision making must be presented to and approved by higher administration before action takes place.

Who is the Boss?

In this game, administration delegates power and authority to the titular "boss," but among the people under her so-called authority is one person who functions as the *real* boss. This usually happens either because the titular "boss" abdicates her authority or because upper level personnel support the "real" boss' power. If the so-called boss attempts to exert authority over the "real" boss, higher authority will countermand her decisions. So we play the game of let's pretend, and the result, once again, is accountability without authority.

Kick the Ego

In situations like *Let's Pretend You Have Power* and *Who is the Boss?,* people in positions of accountability often feel insecure and threatened. They respond like the man who, having been chewed out by his boss, hits his wife, who spanks the child, who kicks the cat. That is, they often take out their frustrations on their co-workers, who have even less power than they do, by making unreasonable demands in order to assert *some* authority and reassure themselves. This situation creates an untenable work environment characterized by uncooperative behaviors, high absenteeism, and poor patient care.

There are other games, such as *You Doctor, Me Handmaiden* and *Six Aids = One RN,* and probably millions more. However, their existence is not nearly as important as the ability of nursing managers to recognize them and define the *real* problems hidden behind them, so that solutions can be formulated. The time has come to quit playing games and get down to the very real business of patient care.

*Reprinted from Nursing Management, ©1982; 13(10):73 with permission from S-N Publications, Inc.

Reality Testing*

CAROL E. CLELAND, R.N., B.S.

Correcting the Overbite

Patrick O'Sullivan resembled a leprechaun with his tufts of white hair, red cheeks, and a softly high-pitched voice. He was 94 years old, 94 pounds heavy, and lived most of his waking hours in mental confusion. With my first few weeks of experience as a nursing student behind me, I was becoming somewhat blasé about the chatter of confused patients. Thus, I heard but didn't hear ". . . Someone's biting me, someone's biting me. . . . Let's go out to dinner today, I'll pay. . . . Where's my overshoes?"

Patrick wasn't assigned to me, but I would stop to pull him up in bed or give him a drink. ". . . How be ye, dearie? Come closer." I leaned closer and he whispered, "Do ya have a bit o' ale?—the water's awful. By the bye, someone's biting me." I reassured him that no one was biting him and asked if apple juice would do.

He continued to chatter about being bitten so I decided to turn him and look, sure the gesture would settle him down. I couldn't believe what I saw. Embedded in his thin buttock was his lower denture. With a red face I showed it to him. "Say, dearie," he responded, "where'd ya find 'em? I've been wondering where they be. Now be a good girl and let the dogs out."

To be honest, I stole a side glance under that bed—no dogs!

Creative Autoclaving

At the end of a hectic Monday in the operating room during my second year in nursing school, I saw a patient have a radioactive substance implanted during surgery. A technician made a dramatic entrance into the OR, shielded in lead—including heavy, long leather lead-filled gloves. Later, when the room and equipment were deemed safe, I was sent to clean, pack, and sterilize the used instruments—but I was not sure what to do with the gloves. It crossed my mind to ask, but the supervisor was not particularly patient at that hour. I decided to go ahead on my own, remembering her frequently repeated words: "I want EVERYTHING clean and sterile."

I wrapped the gloves ever so carefully in a large wrapper, sealed it with tape, labeled the contents, and put them in the autoclave.

When the autoclave was opened, I found I had created two solid six-inch high statues of hands—the original gloves were gone forever. How was I to know that lead melts under extreme heat and leather doesn't do well either!? I'll spare you the details of the discovery scene but those "hands" still grace the supervisor's desk—as bookends.

How to Bag a Dear

Babies never seemed to be born at consistent and steady intervals—either the labor rooms were filled or there were no patients. It was during a quiet time that my supervisor, who did not care for the trend toward more "meaningful educational experiences," assigned housekeeping chores—such as dusting, refolding already folded linen, and restocking the physicians' dressing rooms with green gowns and trousers. One day I was assigned to do all three. Before I completed them, however, a woman was rushed in who seemed ready to deliver. I became involved with her care but it was a false alarm. Instead of returning to finish the housekeeping chores, I spent the time listening to the patient talk about her doctor. "He's such a dear," she said. "So unflappable . . . such a dry sense of humor."

Later an urgent call went back to the dressing room for her obstetrician to hurry. Within seconds he came hopping down the hall. Yes, hopping—a large cotton laundry bag tied around his waist. As he passed me he puffed, "There aren't any pants in the dressing room."

My meeting with the supervisor that followed could have been classified as a "meaningful educational experience."

Some Things Need Footnotes

And then there was the time I ran the college Student Health Center. At the weekly department head staff meetings, our elderly dean would delicately express nervous concerns about other schools reporting great increases in social and health problems.

Weekly, I would confirm his fear that we were indeed part of those statistics, but hasten to reassure him that we had a competent staff and good rapport with the students. I frequently invited him to visit. He'd agree but never show up.

One day following an outbreak of hepatitis, 20 students crowded into our small quarters awaiting injections of gamma globulin. The dean called to say he needed a shot, too. I doubted this, knowing his lack of exposure to students, but thought it would be a good opportunity for him to visit. So I told him to come over and we'd talk about it.

I saw three more students and had just finished with John, who was 6'2" tall and weighed 200 pounds.

"I didn't even feel it," he bragged.

"That's good," I said. "Pull up your trousers and send in the next person." I turned away to record on his chart, then looked around to say good-bye. He was reaching to open the door. "Hey, John! Hold on a minute—your pants are still down." He started to turn, ashen and obviously about to faint. I ran to catch him but he was too heavy so I tried to cushion his fall and we ended up on the floor, with John on top of me. But then, I couldn't budge him. I called out for help. The door opened. The dean had arrived.

Listen Here!*

VIRGINIA MOORE DeWEES, R.N.

One thing they never told me in nursing school was how to wear a stethoscope gracefully. Stethoscopes come in basic black, and assorted colors and in two lengths—very long and very short. Wearing one is like sporting a necklace without a clasp. It's only a matter of time until a vigorous nod sends it slithering to the floor. This usually happens in front of a patient, who then experiences the onset of acute skepticism. It rarely happens in the nurses' station where one can risk carotid compression by leaving it on or whiplash by trying to remove it in a hurry.

I've tried to make a healthy adjustment to this albatross. I've slung it horizontally around my neck like a damp bath towel. I've carried it doubled up in one hand like a recalcitrant Slinky toy. I've let it flap in the breeze like a wilted antenna. I was wondering if the FDA would consider a ban on stethoscopes until I noticed a doctor casually slip one into the pocket of his sports jacket. There it remained, subdued and convenient. Thinking my problem was solved, I tucked a stethoscope into my uniform pocket and sauntered into a patient's room. Nonchalantly, I whipped out the stethoscope—along with pencil, pen, bandage scissors, comb, and nail file.

Nonchalantly, I slipped out of the room, dragging my poise behind me.

Lately I've begun aversion therapy. I leave stethoscopes on bedside tables where they can snake their way around water pitchers, and patients can while away hours fighting through chrome and rubber to fetch a Kleenex.

Meanwhile, I'm working on a device that will fold stethoscopes up like metal tape measures, a uniform with a gigantic pocket, and a doctor to carry my stethoscope.

What They Don't Teach You in Nursing School*

SUZANNE GOLIGHTLY, R.N., B.S.N.

I've finally figured out what keeps the nurses at our hospital flexible: *constant change*. I've adjusted to new and different phone companies and phones, test requisition forms, charting systems, job titles, IV tubing, syringes, drug delivery systems, and patient-care delivery systems.

After assimilating all these changes, I thought my flexibility quotient was pretty high. Then they changed the floor numbers. One day the labs were on two; the next day they were on three. The cafeteria used to be on ground, but not any more; ground is the first floor now. After fifteen years at this hospital, suddenly I don't know where anything is.

The rule about change and flexibility is only one of the unwritten laws they didn't tell us about in nursing school. Here are a few more.

A watched IV bottle never empties. IVs finish only when you aren't in the room. I've learned to loiter outside the door and peek through the slit at the hinges. That way, the instant the bottle empties, I can run in and change it before air enters the tubing.

Unwatched stethoscopes disappear. I have two possible explanations for this phenomenon. First, limp stethoscopes eventually make their way to a stethoscope graveyard (next-door to the elephants' graveyard). Or, some sly resident has a fetish for black tubing and silver earplugs.

Semiprivate rooms make more work. Does the following scenario sound familiar? Patient A asks for a pain pill. You trot down the hall, get the pill, and trot back to deliver it. Only then does patient B ask for his pain pill. I've concluded that roommates decide ahead of time when *not* to want the same thing. You disagree?

Well, next time take two of something to save a trip, and watch patient B say, "Pain pill? Why would I want that?"

Admitting puts patients with the same name in the same room as often as they can. Maybe they think this will save us some time, since both patients can answer one question at the same time. The potential for humor is certainly there. But it can wear thin—Helen Smith in bed one can laugh off the shave prep meant for Helen Smyth in bed two. But her enema?

The patients get food while the staff gets leftovers. Try to find any of the patients' gourmet selections in the staff cafeteria. Their leftover meat and vegetables become our soup of the day. I must admit, though, that the Jell-O looks the same. You have to stab it with your spoon to discover how much more *durable* ours is.

Each hospital has a favorite food it uses in everything. Ours is pineapple. I've found it underneath sculpted mounds of mashed potatoes and balanced on top of spaghetti. In case the patients mutter about truckload specials, have a lecture on the need to balance food groups ready at a moment's notice.

The sweetest patients break every rule. I caught one otherwise delightful patient switching our light bulbs for higher-watt bulbs of her own. If I'd let her get any further, the lampshades would have started to melt. The only solution is to search everyone's luggage for contraband.

I've decided that the faster the orientees learn our institution's unwritten rules, the quicker they'll become effective members of our health team. So I'm on my way to give them a lecture on finding contraband in 15 seconds or less. If only I could find my unit that fast. It used to be on three. Is it on four now?

Things Our Instructors Never Told Us*

KATHLEEN POOLE, R.N., B.S.N.

Our nursing school instructors did a first-class job of teaching us everything we needed to know about patient care. After graduation, we could operate respirators; pinch-hit in the operating room or the intensive care unit (ICU); deliver a baby in an emergency; and deliver encouraging words to a worried patient. I was convinced my instructors hadn't left a stone unturned—until I got out into the real nursing world.

My first few months on a medical/surgical unit were a series of rude awakenings. Take lunch hours, for instance. My first day on the job, I learned that nurses *don't* take lunch hours. If we're lucky, we take lunch *half-hours*. Imagine my dismay the first time I spent half of my lunch half-hour standing in the cafeteria line and most of the other half of my lunch half-hour trying to find a place to sit.

If only our instructors had told us that full lunch hours were a *myth*. Then we could've prepared better—perfected our food inhaling techniques or come up with a variety of excuses for why we were late getting back to work.

My second rude awakening was learning that I wasn't the whiz kid I thought I was when it came to dealing with difficult patients. Take Mr. Smith, for example. *He* wasn't letting a little thing like an appendectomy keep *him* down. When I found him snuggling under the covers with a female visitor, all the appropriate responses I'd memorized flew out the window.

Or take Mr. Jones, who wasn't about to let a case of hemorrhoids ruin *his* sense of humor. Just for laughs, he used his telephone to call the code team to an empty room. I stormed into his room to give him a piece of my mind, but his ebullient high spirits went undampened. Unlike me, who found myself on the receiving end of a full urinal. "Catch," he called merrily, as he heaved the urinal in my direction. Only one

response was appropriate in that situation, but not having lightening-quick reflexes, I missed the catch.

Then there was Mr. Ward, a 250-pound patient who fainted in a 4×4-foot shower stall when the only other staff member not on his lunch break was a 65-year-old, 95-pound ward clerk. (*Together*, we didn't weigh as much as the patient.) We could respond to that situation in one of two ways, we decided—either by bursting into tears or trying to move the patient. We chose the latter, and like two ants moving a boulder, we managed to get Mr. Ward into a wheelchair and back into bed.

I wasn't prepared for difficult visitors, either. I was stunned when a patient's mother threatened to "beat me to a pulp," and if that didn't do the trick, to "wrap me around a telephone pole." (She was angry because I'd told the doctor that I thought she might be tampering with her son's I.V.) The next day, though, instead of carrying out her threats, she apologized, saying she'd only been kidding. Some sense of humor.

Another thing our instructors failed to mention was what a barrel of laughs some doctors can be. I once walked into a patient's room, and the doctor, not known for his sunny disposition, said, "Look what the cat dragged in." Another time, when I asked him if he needed help making rounds, he said, "No—why don't you just go play in a busy street, instead?" Since I was quite speechless, I didn't even try for an appropriate response. I simply smiled *inappropriately* and left the room.

But not all doctors are insulting—some are even complimentary. That is, if you consider a proposition a compliment. I was making rounds with one young doctor, and we stopped to check on an elderly, unresponsive patient. When the doctor finished examining the patient, he grabbed my arm and asked me to go out with him that night.

"No thanks," I said. "I'm so tired, I'm just going home and go to bed."

"Alone?" he said. "You wouldn't have to go to bed alone if I were there."

So I took a firmer approach, but the doctor kept persisting. Finally, the "unresponsive" patient opened her eyes and snapped:

"Oh, for crying out loud, say 'yes' so I can get some sleep."

I'd hardly begun getting used to the idiosyncrasies of patients, visitors, and doctors, when I stumbled over still another unturned stone—hospital red tape. I discovered that a computer ran the hospital, and although the computer had a low tolerance for human error, it had a way of making its own mistakes and then pinning the blame on us. To order even a cotton swab from central supply, we had to fill out special color-coded forms and feed them into the computer. Then, if we somehow got colostomy bags instead of cotton swabs, our penance was to spend still more time filling out forms and punching buttons.

I learned that transferring a patient from room 201 to room 202 on the same unit is harder than transferring him to another hospital—or another planet. The computer arranges transfers, too, and a nurse has to spend at least an hour filling out forms and *replacing* (not just revising) the patient's cards and charts.

Our instructors also forgot to mention how exhausted a young, able-bodied nurse gets working on a unit staffed only with older, less able-bodied nurses. (Especially if the unit happens to be orthopedics—which should be staffed with former Olympic champions.) Or, what happens to your sanity when you float to three different units 3 days in a row. A friend of mine floated from her regular unit, pediatrics, to the ICU. Three months later, when she developed an ulcer, she swore it was from the 8 hours she'd spent in the ICU.

Now that I've been around a bit, I realize our instructors simply couldn't tell us everything. But some of the things they omitted were pleasant surprises—like unexpected gifts to be opened, one by one. Like how happy and proud we feel when a patient gets better; when a doctor says, "Well done"; or when a supervisor says, "When I got you, I got a good deal." And I've discovered something else—the rude awakenings come less often, but the surprise packages never stop.

Hospital Equipment*

ROY BLAIR, R.N.

"Would you do Mr. Brown's warm saline compresses at ten o'clock?" my team leader asked, "You'll have to use the hot plate in the kitchen, the warming cupboard is on the blink."

"You should have been here last week," she went on. "That fool cupboard turned itself on so high that the saline started to boil in the bottles, and when you opened the door and the cold air hit them, they popped their caps at you. We not only had to used a folded towel to open the door, but we had to remember to duck. We forgot to warn Joan and you should see the shiner she has. Had to send her home under sedation," she added.

"Is there anything I should know about the hot plate?" I asked.

"It works," she answered. "Just turn it on about a year before you want anything hot."

I placed the bottle of saline in a pan of water on the hot plate and switched it on.

"Hospital equipment," I mused, and stared out the window . . .

Now if you people will just follow me," the head nurse said, "I'll show you around the ward." The group of students, including myself, followed her down the hall.

"The beds here are all electric," she went on. "Number 16 is empty; we'll go in here and I'll show

* Reproduced with permission from The Canadian Nurse/L'infirmiere canadienne, ©1982; 78(7):46–48.

you how they work." We crowded in behind her and stood staring at the bed.

"This is where it all happens," she said, pointing to a set of small switches on the side. "Now to raise the bed you use this switch." She flicked it to demonstrate, and nothing happened. She stared at the stationary object and muttered something I didn't quite catch.

"This switch raises the head," she continued undaunted; again nothing happened.

"We have been having some problems," she stated; "nevertheless they are very good beds." She patted the bed and, as if in response, the entire structure began a slow descent towards the floor. We all stood and watched in silence as the bed moved down as far as it would go, and then with a little click, stopped.

"Well," the head nurse said, "you'll get used to them; now let's go down to the utility room."

She was wrong. I would never get used to them. I could never remember which bed in which room performed in what way. In some rooms the bed only went up and not down; in other rooms, the reverse was true. The head could be raised on a number of beds but only the foot on others; some of them flatly refused to do anything at all.

The first thing I did learn was that a bed maker could get a real shock, hence morning care was usually punctuated by small squeals, muffled shrieks and muttered curses. The staff wasn't alone in getting shocks from the beds; the patients got their share also. In some cases, it was an instant cure for immobility. Patients, who only the day before required a lot of verbal support, not to mention three able-bodied orderlies just to sit upright, suddenly found themselves standing straight and tall in the middle of the room. Not until midnight would they return to bed and even then with the greatest reluctance.

A few of the beds operated independently, moving up or down, flipping up their head or foot at random. A patient could be resting flat and quiet one minute; then the head of the bed would suddenly fly up, summersaulting him into an hysterical heap at the foot. No, I never did get used to those beds.

I first encountered the stove when a patient asked me for warm milk. Placing the pan on the large left front element, I switched it on to medium. It hissed and then produced some of the most beautiful blue sparks I have ever seen, but no heat. I tried the element

behind it, nothing again. Then the one beside it, with the same results, and finally the right front. Although I tuned it to medium, it obliged by turning a bright, angry red. The first element, which was turned off, hissed and made with the blue sparks again; I countered by jumping and spilling the milk. I found out later that the large element was considered eccentric but harmless. The performance of the two back elements depended on a variety of things such as mood swings, atmospheric pressure and, as one staff member suggested, "whether I wear my cap or not." The remaining element worked on high no matter what its switch was set at; it seems element and dial simply could not agree.

The fridge was in the medicine room. This room, in keeping with the criteria of most hospitals, was about the size of a pay toilet, but not as convenient. The fridge was hip height, which meant bending almost double to get anything out of it. The door, when opened, cleared the floor by about two inches—just the right height to take the top off your shoes. Regardless, opening the door presented another problem: when open, there wasn't enough space for you to stay in the room. This meant that as the door opened the nurse backed out of the room, and when the door was fully opened she stepped back in again. This was only the beginning, as the next move was to get down far enough to see in.

The first day I faced the machine, I knew what had to be done. In the best nursing tradition, bent from the knees and keeping my back straight, I descended to fridge level. My left knee pushed everything on the top shelf into a jumble at the back, while my right knee slid into the open freezer compartment. When I mentioned this to my instructor, she suggested that I stand sideways to the fridge, bend, and then turn my head at a sharp right angle. However, as my head was attached in the normal manner and not on a swivel as hers was, I stuck with the frozen knee method.

A few of the staff preferred to stand in the medicine room doorway, open the fridge door towards them, then bend over it and peer, ostrich fashion, into the interior. This, however, left them open to any number of rude comments, not to mention flying rubber bands. I still think my method was the best and I have an arthritic knee to prove it.

The second day on the ward, I met the ice machine. This contraption was referred to by the staff as "Ice Machine," and was given the male gender.

"He wet all over my shoe," I heard one nurse complain and naturally thought she was referring to a patient.

Ice Machine was located in a small dark alcove off the main corridor. He stood five feet high and was nearly as broad; originally constructed in stainless steel, he had degenerated to a sad looking gun-metal grey. He was equipped with a large, hinged flap door in the front and had a perpetual puddle of water at his feet. "Stress incontinence," I thought, making a snap diagnosis.

Ice Machine's door was hinged at the top and designed so that it would not stay open unless held. This presented a problem as I had a pitcher in one hand and a scoop in the other. I solved this by propping the cold metal door against my shoulder, leaving my hands free. Ice Machine rewarded my resourcefulness by dropping the largest piece of ice he could make onto the back of my hand.

He was a night person. He stood in his alcove all day, muttering to himself; however, during the 12-to-8 shift, he was in his element. He coughed and shook and rattled his door. He put together the biggest pieces of ice possible and dropped them from a great height, while the smaller cubes were tossed out into the hall with gay abandon. One of his most disconcerting noises was a long, shuddering, asthmatic wheeze, followed by a series of rattles and ending by a bang of his door. Then, with the first light of dawn, he subsided into a generalized grumble and started reserving his strength for the next midnight shift.

Staff were always careful about what they said in front of this machine because they never knew what his reaction would be. One day, a new staff member referred to Ice Machine as "that piece of geriatric junk," The next time she went to get ice, he dropped his door on her foot.

Ice Machine was a seasonal person. He loved the winter and hated the summer. As the days got progressively warmer, he went into a decline, producing a small amount of ice, which was pitted and soft. Finally, on the hottest day of the year, with a little rattling sigh he turned himself off; Ice Machine met his end. We went to another floor for ice after that.

The water in the basin started to boil and I came back to the present. Lifting the now warm bottle of saline out of its bath, I started across the kitchen, but paused in front of the ice machine.

"Young," I thought, eyeing it critically, "too new and shiny, no character, but maybe in another ten years, who knows." I hurried away while the saline was still warm.

Elevator Excursions*

TANYA M. SUDIA ROBINSON, M.N., R.N.

Hospitals and elevators go hand-in-hand. In order to successfully navigate the hospital terrain, you must recognize that elevators have their own lingo, negotiation strategies, and patterns of dysfunction. Consider this a crash course in how to survive your next elevator excursion.

Let's start with elevator lingo. "MASH 12" is not a new M.A.S.H. unit, nor the twelfth version of the movie. Instead, "MASH 12" is elevatorese for "Please push the 12th floor button." When speaking elevatorese, single words become sentences that have nothing to do with healthcare. For example, the elevator doors open and someone asks, "Down?" This person is not interested in your emotional state; they simply want to know which direction the elevator is headed.

Elevators also have their own rules of etiquette. You must learn to follow these rules or suffer the consequences. For instance, when the doors open and the elevator appears full, do not use your social graces to wait for the next one. Instead, squeeze on. Others will do the same. It does not matter that the weight or person limit has been exceeded. Nor does it matter that the weight limit alarm sounds. You will eventually block out the sound just like the rest of the passengers do.

In addition to learning the elevator lingo and etiquette, you must learn the Art of Negotiation. Invariably, at some point in time you will end up in the back corner of a very crowded elevator and need to exit on the 8th floor; the elevator doors will have opened and shut before you get a polite sentence out and you'll still be in the back of the elevator. Instead, be direct and yell "Coming Out!" This is what is known as a winning negotiation strategy.

The ultimate elevator experience is getting stuck on the elevator which, according to Murphy's Law, only happens when your stress level is sky-high and it is the hottest day of the year. To make hospital life even more interesting, the elevator I was stuck on included 14 other people. Most interesting was the man standing next to me. I was looking down and noticed that his ankles were chained together. As my eyes slowly moved upward, I saw the prison name imprinted on his pant leg. I dared to let my eyes walk upward to his hands and was relieved to see that they were cuffed. Of course, I next looked up to see his face only to have him give me a sly smile. What could I do but smile back and wonder how many murders he had committed and if I'd be next! Meanwhile, his escort guard was panicking with the rest of the crew.

As luck would have it, the outside temperature was 95 degrees that day. Since the air conditioning unit turns off whenever the elevator gets stuck, the inside elevator temperature had to be at least 105 degrees. As you hear those around shouting for help and swearing that they will faint, you calmly remember the CODE phone. (These are found in side panel boxes in most elevators.) The problems begin when the telephone operator asks you which elevator you are on. Since the number is painted on the outside door of the elevator, and you are stuck on the inside, you cannot answer that question intelligently. So, give the next most logical answer, "The one that is stuck."

Once you are rescued from the elevator, you promise yourself to take the stairs the next time. That is, until you are on the first floor and remember that you work on the 14th floor. Soon you are back to riding elevators, only to get stuck again.

But, this time you get stuck with a savvy nurse rather than a prisoner. Like all smart nurses, her pockets are full of survival equipment. She promptly pulls out her bandage scissors and pries the doors apart while a co-worker forces the doors open. A word of caution: since elevators often get stuck between floors, realize that you will have to take quite a step up to exit.

---

*Reprinted from Point of View, ©1992; 29(1):17 with permission from Ethicon, Inc.

There are two more hazards to getting stuck in the elevator. One is that you are not prepared for emergencies. For instance, you are the only health-care personnel in an elevator with a pregnant woman. She happens to be in active labor and starts to fall to the floor. You naturally presume that the man with her is actually with her. It turns out that he merely blocked her fall to the ground. Better yet, she does not speak a word of English and you have never delivered a baby.

The second hazard is that getting stuck will cause you to be late for a meeting or some other significant life event. In one case, I ended up late for my exit interview. When I arrived, the interviewer stated, "You are late! I expected you twenty minutes ago. I don't know if we can fit you in." If this happens, calmly remember that personnel employees do not have nursing assessment skills. She does not notice that your breathing is shallow and rapid, or that you are tachycardic, hypertensive, and diaphoretic. One thing is for certain: you will not forget your last day there nor will you have any regrets about leaving.

If life should become boring at your hospital, go to your nearest elevator and ride it for awhile. I guarantee that you will eventually experience an excursion worth writing home about.

Telesco's Laws*

MARIA TELESCO

1. All the I.V.'s are at the other end of the hall.

2. A physician's ability is inversely proportional to his availability.
   Corollary to #2:
   A physician's availability is inversely proportional to his ability.

3. There are two kinds of adhesive tape: that which won't stay on and that which won't come off.

4. Everybody wants a pain shot at the same time.

5. Everybody who didn't want a pain shot when you were passing out pain shots wants one when you are passing out sleeping pills.

6. Whenever a mistake is made in the pay checks, it is always in their favor.

7. Staffing by acuity means they can take away nurses when *they* think you have too many, but they cannot give you more nurses when *you* think you have too few.

Telesco's Hypothesis Concerning Nursing Administration's Theorem of Staffing:
   If two people ask for the same day off and only one can have it, give it to neither, as it is preferable to have two nurses miserable than to have one nurse happy.

If Oliver North Taught Hospital Administration*

MARY B. MALLISON, R.N.

"This place makes St. Elsewhere look like the Mayo Clinic!" quipped an exasperated head nurse the other day. Her reaction reflects the tenor of thousands of answers we've received both from our June Nurse-Work survey and from Priscilla Scherer's probe of frontline nurses' reactions to the shortage.

Many of these nurses aimed their most blistering criticism at hospital administrators. The combination of the nurses' comments, plus a summer overdose of Iran-contra hearings, caused our eyes to glaze over when we looked up college catalogs to see what hospital administrators actually are being taught these days. Here's what we thought we saw in those catalogs.†

Hospital PR 201: How to pretend St. Elsewhere is the St. Regis. Prerequisite: *Redecorating Lobbies and Administrative Suites.*

Creative Budgeting 301: How to lay off hospital personnel and persuade Nursing to pick up the slack, while at the same time making Nursing feel it has power because it didn't have to lay off anyone.

Toughing It Out 302: How to keep perpetually short of supplies as a way to convince employees that if the finances aren't there for supplies, they certainly aren't there for raises, either.

The Swiss Switch (also called *Oliver North at the Bank*): How to encourage the nursing department to cut nursing management positions so you can use the money "saved" to create more hospital administrative positions without adding to the overall bottom line. Prerequisite: *Why Administrators Must Reproduce: The Power of Numbers 201.*

Sartorial Etiquette 101: Required first semester. Teaches the value of the three-piece suit (for men) and the silk blouse (for women). Clearly delineates your role as administrative, so that staff won't ask you to help move beds or mop up spills.

The QA Audit as Filibuster (also called *Paperhanging 202*): Known in Washington parlance as the Limited Hangout. How to talk your way through JCAH and state regulatory agency visits by first burying the visitors in documents and then showing them only what you want them to see. Essential to keep Nursing and other departments so preoccupied with trying to correct their deficiencies in documentation that they don't have the energy to plan an end run.

Art Appreciation—That Certain Smile: An in-depth study of the *Mona Lisa.* Features closed-circuit-TV role-playing, during which student is asked embarrassing questions. Teaches the art of the enigmatic smile and frozen silence, especially useful when discussions of "how much did the hospital earn last year?" begin.

Hospital Marketing 201 (Shifting the Blame): Teaches the hidden value in making sure all employees are run through a brief hospitality course. It may not change their behavior but, thereafter, they are more susceptible to accepting blame if patients continue to choose other hospitals instead of your own.

Pretending to Listen: How to look directly at a nurse who insists Dr. X is dangerous. You know you won't do anything about Dr. X because he admits too many patients to this hospital. Course teaches you to maintain sympathetic eye contact while mentally tying trout flies. See related course, *How to Encourage Complaining as a Substitute for Action.*

Family Dynamics: How to convince staff "We're all one big happy family here," while announcing unilateral decision to cut benefits.

Divide and Conquer 402: How to keep knowledge as power by limiting or thwarting communication between departments. Teaches how to sow doubts about Department A's truthfulness or competence in the minds of Department B. See related course below.

Isolate and Destroy 401: How to convince the VP for Nursing that you, her CEO, are the only person she should trust. Meanwhile, you discourage her involvement in any nursing organization or community activity that, by widening her base of support, could make her harder to fire when the time comes.

AS TIME GOES BY

Though it may seem imperceptible on a daily basis, change is ever occurring. The challenge to nursing is to stay flexible and resilient in adapting to the increasing pace of societal and technological advances.

Because nurses are the largest segment of health care providers, they hold the richest promise for answers to today's myriad health care problems. Nurses should not fear the process of change, but rather accept it as an opportunity to reassess their strengths for the coming century.

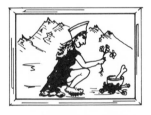

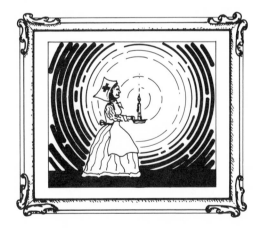

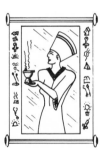

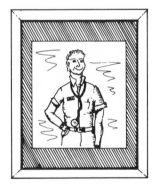

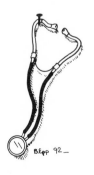

Hickory Dickory . . .
A Fable for Our Times*

JOAN M. RINEHART, R.N., PH.D.

It was a hot sultry morning and Florence Nursenmouse wished she hadn't agreed to do this interview with Art Bookvole. Besides, she was very busy because some of the other mice were unable to work this morning. Art was asking her another question . . .

ART: Why do you think the American Rat Association set up this award to honor a white mouse such as you?

FLO: Well, you must understand that mice like me are devoted to helping the rats and have been for years, so they may want to reward mice that work with them, perhaps to encourage others to follow the traditional way. In case you're unaware of it, not all the mice feel this way any more.

ART: You got the award because you're loyal?

FLO: I hope I got it because I'm good at my work. Even though the rats have bigger and sharper teeth, I can gnaw just as well, given time—except for the big jobs, of course.

ART: Don't the rats resent your chewing into their territory, so to speak?

FLO: Oh, no. They need me for the little places they can't get to, and I'd *never* try to do the really big jobs. Besides, there are so many of the smaller jobs to do, the rats could never handle all of them. There are more of us mice than there are rats, you know, so the rats do depend on us.

ART: Speaking of numbers, I hear that the white mice like you are decreasing in numbers and may even become extinct. Is that true?

FLO: Well . . . yes, we used to be more prolific. Then our reproduction rate dropped off and is still continuing to drop. We're trying to reverse the trend, and some of the rats are helping, but we just haven't had much success yet.

ART: I heard that it may be because you're not adapting to change—genetically, that is.

FLO: You've been talking to those gray field mice, haven't you? They think we're sick because we're white. Well, they may have mutated to longer tails and bigger teeth, but they still won't survive.

ART: Ah . . . I did talk to Lucy Quinline about this. She and many of the other field mice do seem to be adapting with sharper, bigger teeth, but they are also increasing in number, they tell me.

FLO: Maybe so, but there are just not enough of them to have a major effect on the breed. Furthermore, they're trying to do rat jobs because of this, and that doesn't make the rats happy; they still have a lot of power, you know.

ART: By the way, what do you think of those very long-tailed mice who have a mania for eating books? There's a large number of them, I hear. Now don't tell me that they're mutants!

FLO: No, of course not. They're just plain crazy. Can you imagine the waste of time—the utter uselessness—of chewing books with no food value? And they're not even chewing their way to food! Now that's not logical or sane.

ART: What do the rats have to say about this?

FLO: The rats don't even worry about them. I guess it's because they stay out of the rats' way, but the rats do agree that it's a waste of time. You should see them! Once they've had a taste of the books, they just won't give them up, even when their teeth grow shorter and more dull.

Did you know, they want *all* of us mice to chew books? They say it would make our tails grow. Now isn't that ridiculous! We need something to strengthen our teeth and to increase our reproduction rate, not give us uselessly long tails.

ART: You don't think they'll be able to make all the mice chew even a few books?

*Reprinted from Nursing Outlook, ©1980; 28(7):432–433 with permission from Mosby Year Book.

FLO: Oh, my goodness, no! Why, those long-tailed creatures can't even agree among themselves on the books we should chew.

It certainly isn't the first time they've had a problem. Look at what a mistake they made when they developed the off-white breed to replace us. They ended up creating stubby-tailed little things with short, dull teeth simply because they put them through the Tooth and Tail Institute much faster than we went through . . . My, the time we waste just training them on the job!

But that's another story. The one thing you must remember is that we white mice are still very much in the majority, and we have strength in our numbers. We will eventually win out. The rest of the mice will see this and come running back. You watch, you'll see how they run.

ART: No, I don't see. If your reproduction rate is steadily dropping, then the others will eventually become the majority. Besides, haven't you heard "You can't go home again"? You really can't go back in time.

FLO: I don't believe that! Are you saying that everything is going to change because the white mice will all be gone? I just can't accept that.

Who would do our jobs? Certainly not the long-tailed book eaters; they don't have the teeth for it. The gray field mice don't want to do what we do, and those little off-white mice with only a stub of a tail could never fill our place—their teeth aren't up to it, either. The fact is, our work will always be there, and there will always be a need for our kind.

ART: Perhaps you mean there will always be need for someone to do the work, but it may not necessarily always be "your kind." Maybe those others will be "running" ahead to something different, not running back to what was.

FLO: You just don't understand. There will always be white mice.

Bandwagons Nursing Has Jumped On—or Off:

A Satire on Some of the Events in the History of Nursing Education*

MARION M. SCHRUM, Ed.D., R.N.

In the course of a career that may, by some standards, be distinguished by length rather than fame, it has been my observation that nursing is somewhat distinctive in its history. Unlike most other professions whose evolutions follow a reasonably straight line, modern nursing's development has been somewhat circuitous, if not downright confusing. Much like the San Francisco tourist on the famed cable car, nurses, particularly nurse educators, have jumped on and clung to the sides of many bandwagons.

The early development of nursing education in this country *was* fairly consistent. Programs evolved from what was essentially a one-year apprenticeship dominated by the needs of the hospital to a three-year program which, in many cases, was still the servant of the hospital's needs. No one paid any attention to Florence Nightingale, who said that a school of nursing should be separately endowed.

All schools were controlled by the hospitals and the "good schools" taught what the National League for Nursing (then known as the National League for Nursing Education) and the state boards of nursing told them to teach. All states ultimately required a licensure examination. Since not all examinations were exactly

*Reprinted from Journal of Professional Nursing, ©1986; 2(4):199–200 with permission from W.B. Saunders Co. and the author. Edited from the original.

alike, a thing called reciprocity developed so nurses could move from state to state. In due time, a national test pool was developed, making migration somewhat easier—except for the paperwork.

Nursing education was fairly clear until a few educators with great vision determined that nursing education could be best served in colleges and universities. While one school was put under the aegis of a university in 1909 at the University of Minnesota, not much happened until 1923 when two collegiate schools were started—one at Yale and the other at what is now known as Case Western Reserve University.

The college and university wagon rumbled along rather slowly; the number of passengers increased only gradually. Note that graduates of both types of schools—hospital and university—wrote the same state board examination, and all of them thought they were graduates of professional schools.

In 1950, a nurse educator hypothesized that by removing all of the repetitive experiences from the diploma programs and placing the programs in community colleges, a vocational (or technical) nurse could be prepared efficiently and effectively. Her research supported her hypothesis, but her audience did not hear the words vocational or technical. That wagon swept across the country full-tilt with a host of passengers. The result? Three types of nursing programs whose graduates take the same state board examination, and whose graduates all consider themselves professionals, even though a recommendation for two levels of nursing practice (vocational and technical) was made in 1923 (the Goldmark Report), in 1950 (the Brown Report), and in 1965 (from the ANA House of Delegates). Today the semantic and conceptual arguments regarding two levels of nursing practice prevail, which is another way of saying that some wagons wear out slowly.

Even in the dust and confusion of these bandwagons, graduate programs did emerge. Most of the early programs prepared nurses for teaching, administration and, in some schools, public health nursing. Before long, educators believed nursing knowledge had expanded sufficiently to justify a clinical major. That struck a sensitive nerve in the hearts of many, and another wagon joined the train. In fact, the idea was so popular that "functional majors" were either disbanded or relegated to minor status. The belief still lingers that if you can do you can teach. That is, of course, in opposition to the old adage that if you can't do it, teach

it, and if you can't teach it, teach how to teach it. Many have realized, however, that administration, for example, is a learned skill, and are hopping back onto the functional major bandwagon.

Post-basic education did not escape its measure of confusion, however. The concept of the nurse practitioner (aren't we all nurse practitioners?) emerged in the 1960s and many people thought that the expanded role would give nurses the opportunity to demonstrate their level of intelligence and add a bit of status in the bargain. This led to six-month, nine-month, 12-month, and even 18-month programs for graduates of two-, three-, and four-year programs. Mathematically, that yields a fair number of combinations (or dyads, if you prefer that term), all leading to the title nurse practitioner. Nursing had again shunned the mainstream of higher education, and left the public behind, interested but confused at the profession's many educational permutations. Only now is there hope that all programs of advanced education should be at the graduate level.

The concept of the unification model is an interesting one, too. Many will recall that in the early days of nursing education in this country, teachers often held a position in the hospital as well—in other words, a dual role. As nursing grew more sophisticated, serving two masters became more difficult. Thus, school of nursing faculty were separate from the hospital staff, and the gap between nursing education and nursing service appeared. Each segment blamed the other for the ills of the system. The unification model has emerged to "remedy" this obvious problem. In other words, faculty and nursing service personnel have dual appointments! Feel like we've come full circle? Now, of course, there is still greater sophistication within the profession, but has the old truism changed? Time will have to provide the answer. A little dip into history might help, too.

The registered nurse seeking a baccalaureate degree also has been the victim of a little wagon-jumping. Remember the days of the blanket credit plus two years of liberal arts? Those days were followed by an equally erroneous assumption that the RN had learned nothing so was given no credit in any form for previous learning (and then we wondered why so many were so angry). Finally, nurse educators decided to measure and validate what had been learned and designed programs that would build on that knowledge. Some educators became so dedicated to the needs of the registered nurse that all kinds of innovative programs emerged. For example, a nurse in Wyoming could get a degree from a school in Maine and never set foot on campus. Amazing! Expedience set aside the richness of the university environment. These programs demonstrated little sensitivity to the long struggle exerted by other educators to bring nursing into the university as a learned discipline, developing sound programs for two- and three-year graduates.

Many nurse educators grew up with the idea that curriculum development wasn't very mysterious. Most agreed that one started with a statement of philosophy that gave direction to the objectives. Add an understanding of learning theory and one was ready to structure a program that was logically organized and internally consistent.

Then came the notion of the conceptual framework. Early on, this notion was fairly simple: one looked at the student, society, and the profession to provide direction to the development of a conceptual framework. Those of us who used the notion in later years got into trouble in the accreditation process— maybe because the basis for our curriculum wasn't "conceptual" enough. Even those of us with a strong background in philosophy had difficulty getting comfortable with the whole idea. Lots of folks must have, however, because the importance of the conceptual framework resulted in its use as a criterion for accreditation.

Some of us never really liked that wagon, so we stuck to the notion that a curriculum should be logically organized and internally consistent. The term conceptual framework, however, had great appeal until someone *really* important said that the whole notion had become clouded and should be abandoned. Some bright folks on the "look at the accreditation process and the criteria" committee must have listened. When the new criteria came out, nowhere could the term conceptual framework be found. More surprising, however, was its replacement. We returned to the notion that a curriculum should be logically organized and internally consistent! So another wagon lost its luster, its wheels, and its passengers, and was replaced by an old-timer that has withstood the test of time and intellectual tinkering.

I'm an Upwardly Mobile Stick-in-the-Mud*

GILLESPIE RICHARDS, R.N., B.A.

Sending a supervisor to a week-long, out-of-state conference has its advantages: for one, she is not at work. However, the cost is just as obvious: she returns filled with new enthusiasm.

Although we grow deposits for renal and biliary calculi in the Midwest, health care is otherwise relatively risk-free. We take few chances and we are unlikely to be in the pace car at the beginning of the race. Here, health care personnel are mostly of the Ozzie and Harriet genre. I am too, actually.

We "caregivers" still call ourselves nurses. The "clients" look more like patients in their faded, open-backed blue gowns, and any concerns we might have about an upsurge of "emerging professionals" demanding their place in the sun takes a back seat to establishing when each of us goes to first and second breaks.

Picture, then, our supervisor as she returns from *California*. Expecting inservices on acupressure and biofeedback, we get new words with old meanings.

Our leader brings back three wonderful new phrases: third-party payment, marketing our product, and the clinical ladder.

As a primary caregiver to my clients, I could practice my tired-but-patient look of expertise. After that I could file for third-party payment.

I admit I've always had a secret desire to carry a beeper and dash off at a run to call the hospital. I'd be an after-hours consultant: "Which nare did I put the NG down the first time? Yes, it was the right, and feel free to call if you have any other questions."

I dream on as she talks about just how this stepping-stone would bring us parity with physicians. Parity with physicians means, I gather, having their hours, their insurance premiums, and their alimony payments. I'm quite sure it doesn't mean having their sailboats.

"Marketing a product" means developing terrific care plans or teaching booklets and then selling them to other hospitals and clinics. Another nurse stays at the bedside while I'm out selling booklets and care plans. And she would be encouraged to aspire to my job while I would be yearning to get back to what I came for in the first place. First, we cheerfully increase the amount of paperwork, and then we become itinerant salesclerks. And this is progress?

Then comes the not-so-good news. She describes her version of the clinical ladder. Even though I'm happy to tell you my credentials—mother of two boys, Sunday school teacher, fourth-grade room mom, BA in English, AD in nursing, staff nurse—I'm worried that some of them may not be seen as steps that go up.

The plan is to have different levels: staff on the first rung, then primary I and II, and finally clinical I and II. Some of us will be grandfathered in. (Why not grandmothered? Why not bigeminy, tertiary, Duke's grade IV?) Still more sobering is the news that we'll have to rack up continuing education credits and attend conferences and workshops. All this to just obtain or maintain.

Will this become a dog-eat-dog world? Taking nurses out of the "hotel costs" of room and board conjures up a scenario of nurses fighting over IV starts and patients accepting bids for auscultations. On early morning rounds, we see our patient hearing that his "caregiver is Nancy, who will be your primary II today." "Thank you," he says softly under his breath, "but I feel more like I need a primary I . . . ."

Fiction fades away as my supervisor comes up for air, but the feeling lingers long after morning conference.

Long, magnificent extension ladders are on order, already en route to this hospital. I am supposed to welcome them. But when I look down I see I am standing on a ladder of my own—an old, well-used, paint-speckled stepladder with only a few rungs. And I have already climbed high enough to see the top and to read the admonition written there: "This is not a step. Do not stand here."

I Never Wear White
After Dark*

PAULINE J. ALLEY, L.P.N.

Nursing has changed me. And I sometimes wonder if it's been for the better. Years ago, before I traded in my dishpan hands and housemaid's knee for sterile gloves and white stockings, I feverishly read every family health guide I could lay my hands on. I watched for every medical disorder in my family members from Achalasia to Zollinger-Ellison syndrome. When either my husband or one of my children complained of "acid-indigestion," I empathetically patted him on the head, rushed to my resource books and developed a home treatment plan which included total "poor-baby" patient care. I worried. I fretted. And when the symptoms passed, only then did I relax and get on with the business of living.

How different now! After working in a hospital for seven years, I find it hard to take my family's minor discomforts seriously. For example, when the alarm blasted at 5:30 a.m. yesterday morning, instead of hearing a "good morning darling" from my husband, who has fallen victim to total body failure at age 38, I was greeted by this: "Oh, I didn't sleep good. My back hurts, my legs ache, my chest feels congested and the two toes I had amputated eight years ago have phantom limb pain." I immediately resented his choice of words. I dislike laymen using those medical terms like phantom pain and congestion and it sent me into a tizzy. I informed him I wasn't on duty until seven a.m. I rushed to the bathroom, closed the door on him and his missing toes and thoroughly enjoyed emptying my bladder.

Complaints such as these have become all too common around our house and I see how I've been handling them recently. Any complaints received before seven a.m. or after 3:30 p.m. are usually ignored. Those I hear on my days off are only discussed the last thirty seconds on my way out the door to go shopping.

Yet even with my new, non-chalant approach to family health care, some aspects of our family life are improving. My children's school attendance has improved remarkably. No longer are the subjective symptoms of "I feel sort of sick to my stomach, can I stay home from school today?" acceptable. "You want a day off, kid? Then vomit within the next ten minutes and I'll write you a note." Only objective symptoms produce excused absences. Open draining wounds, hematomas and hives fall into this category. The kids are getting the point. They know now that they have to run a fever or run to school.

And once at school, they usually stay there. The only way home is via ambulance. I used to receive at least two calls a week during working hours from Mr. Porter, the grade school principal about my ten-year old. "Mrs Alley," he would begin. "Bernadette is complaining of pain from her temples and across her forehead with some pressure pain on top of her head." After leaving work a number of times (which in a hospital is a major feat in itself) and having the child checked by the pediatrician, I was ready for the next phone call. I only had a two-day wait before talking with Mr. Porter again. This time he was instructed to give her a glass of milk, a one-half hour break in sick bay and a return to her fifth-grade math class. Diagnosis? Tension headache. Problem resolved.

I searched my soul for a while to find the reasons why my family used me as their professional scapegoat. I think I've learned a couple of things I was doing that led to their myriad complaints. Here's what I don't do anymore.

No longer do I talk about my work at home. It's such an easy habit to fall into. Incisions, drainage tubes, incontinency all have a gastro-intestinal effect on unprepared innocents. I once explained the colostomy procedure to three of my teenagers. I thought it might help them if they ever took a creative writing class. Two of them had the "runs" for three days and the third became impacted. None to this day will use plastic sandwich bags. For them, ignorance is bliss.

* Reprinted with permission from Journal of Nursing Care, ©1981; 14(2):16–17.

Now I discourage them from seeing me at work. There was a time that on the holidays I worked, I invited them for lunch in the cafeteria with me. A real treat for them, an embarrassing situation for me. At first they didn't recognize the sweet, gentle expression on my face, my salt and pepper hair topped by my cap of dignity. They gawked at me. "Is that really you Mom?" they said in front of my co-workers who were about to nominate me "Working Mother of the Year." "Is there anything wrong, dah-h-lings?" I managed to blurt out. "Yes," they replied. "When you go shopping, will you buy some Aspirins and band-aids?" Trying to downplay the question, I assured them there must be these necessary items in the medicine cabinet. They were quick to inform me and the rest of my Unit that we had been out of aspirin since New Year's Day and it's too hard to use kleenex and a piece of scotch tape on a cut "like I told them to do."

I've also learned not to mix business with pleasure. My husband and I have noticed immediate rewards from my new rule. When I talked "shop" at home he used to feel he was making love to Resusci-Annie. No longer do I count respirations or take a radial pulse for on-the-spot research of sexercise. Sex has become a non-nursing function. Who cares if it dilates the coronary arteries, anyways?

Yep, nursing has changed me. It's changed my family, too. When I question whether it's been a change for the better, all I have to do is look around. I don't see many ace bandages being used. There's no hot water bottles or Pepto-Bismal in sight. Whoops, I hear someone coughing! It's almost 8 p.m. I have to dash and change my uniform. I never wear white after dark.

My Love Affair with Uniforms*

MARY JANE JANOWSKI, R.N., B.S.N.

No self-respecting nurse would ever admit to being attracted to the profession by, of all things, WEARING A UNIFORM. I won't go so far as to say that was what attracted me, but back in the summer of '73, when I tore into my eagerly awaited letter of acceptance to nursing school, I was really looking for the uniform order sheet.

Visions of parading around my neighborhood in crisp, immaculate Nightingalehood, inspiring awe in even the most casual of passersby, sent me reeling with eager anticipation. A few weeks later my ensemble was complete: light blue pinstriped dress with white bib insert (school emblem in place on the cuffed sleeve), gleaming white (sensible) shoes, white support hose, Timex watch with "sweep second hand," stethoscope, blue cardigan sweater, and of course, the *pièce de résistance*—starched white cap with lofty twin peaks pointing heavenward.

My excitement suffered a minor setback when my class schedule arrived. The first clinical meeting was to take place at the college. NO UNIFORMS. What's one more week on the sands of time (sigh)? The major setback came at the first class. Miss Jackson, associate professor, department of nursing, sternly proclaimed, "NEVER is any part of your uniform to be worn in your home, on the street, on the bus, or anywhere other than within the confines of your clinical unit. Any part of your uniform that is not carried to your unit in a clean, plastic bag will be considered CONTAMINATED." From that moment on, living my fantasy of drinking in the world's response to my being a student nurse consisted of playing "dress up" with my two-year-old, and even then, only after I had made her promise to never tell Miss Jackson.

As graduation approached, it seemed masochistic to wait any longer. I went shopping for an adequate supply of WHITE uniforms, paying close attention to practicality as well as style. Fit was crucial because 1975's high hemlines were sure to become a liability as I stooped to check urine outputs and knelt to snatch life-saving equipment from the innermost reaches of crash carts. My uniforms had to have enough pockets to hold pens, penlights, clamps, and scissors; and ample lapels for appropriate display of school pin and name tag. My image of professionalism demanded traditional tailoring—no trendy empire waists or bell-bottomed pantsuits would ever compromise the efficiency of my working wardrobe.

Since I had often seen nurses wearing their uniforms outside the hospital, I decided to risk contamination and wear my uniform as I walked to work. It was wonderful. The summer sun reflecting off all that white made heads turn from every direction. It took a few minutes to realize that most of those heads were male. Many of them were speaking to me: "Nurse, I'm sick." "Nurse, take my pulse." "Nurse, I bet you know how to make me feel better." "I always wanted to (bleep) a nurse." Was this what Miss Jackson meant by contamination?

Having sustained another burst bubble, I began carrying my uniform to work, at least in warm weather. As this became more of a nuisance with each passing day, I began to see the value of pantsuits. They did seem to attract less attention on the street, and also proved ideal on the med-surg floors. Pantsuits with long tunics and well-fitted pants were marvelous in terms of worry-free bending and reaching. When made of ventilated fabrics, they were the epitome of cool comfort. I often worked in pediatrics, so it wasn't long before I recognized the importance of reading the fabric care labels. (Scotchgard and Z'out became household words.) But above all, I was enjoying recognition as a nurse, at least by my fellow employees and my patients (the only people to whom it was really important anyway).

Just as I began to feel a new sense of "maturity" about uniforms, my career took an unexpected turn. I was offered a job in obstetrics, in the newly created neonatal intensive care unit. Suddenly all my tediously accumulated uniform sense became superfluous as I realized that I was about to don SCRUBS. That's what all those superskilled persons in ORs wear! Imagine scurrying down to the cafeteria for a quick bite between umbilical cannulations and having heads turn with respect as the hospital fluorescence radiated off all that OR green. This was more excitement than even I'd dreamed of.

Well, as any nurse who's ever dealt with hospital linen supplies knows, scrub dresses come in two sizes—3 and 56. Anything in between has already been hoarded. If you're of average height, there is a chance that someday you might find a dress that fits acceptably. If that happens, grab it and a size 3; cut the size 3 into patches to repair the dress. If you're six feet tall like I am, go back to your white wardrobe, wear the bottom halves of your better-fitting pantsuit uniforms, pull the waist cinches out of the size 3 scrubs, and complete your ensemble by wearing the now shapeless greens as tunics. Voila! The best of both worlds! I may have looked ridiculous, but I was able to do my job in cool, clean comfort.

As my nursing career expanded to occasionally include less traditional settings, I became enamored of another kind of professional garb—THE LAB COAT. As a part of my baccalaureate program I worked in a hypertension screening project, and for a few months was again proud to be recognized outside the hospital as a health professional. It wasn't until a most delightful octogenarian asked me if I thought it was time for another blue rinse that I began to question just how much anything that I wore had to do with nursing.

All of us in the nursing profession are most fortunate to live and work in 1983 when flexibility in uniform codes has made the range of individual expression virtually unbounded.

November, 1982, brought welcome news, this time by telephone. I had become assistant editor of *AJN*. Visions of parading around my neighborhood in crisp, impeccably tailored BUSINESS SUITS, inspiring awe in even the most casual of passersby . . . .

The More Things Change . . .*

EDITH P. LEWIS, R.N., M.N., F.A.A.N.

I last practiced hospital nursing in the '40s. At that time the typical equipment for a patient unit included a hospital bed with a Gatch frame that could be hand-cranked up and down at head and knee; a bedside stand, usually with one drawer and a towel rack attached to the back; and an over-the-bed table with a top that lifted up to reveal an inner compartment. The bedside stand was always positioned flat against the wall, out of any reasonable reach of its presumed user.

Now, 40 years later, I've been hospitalized twice, with varying degrees of incapacity. During those four decades, antibiotics and steroids have been discovered, hearts have been transplanted, and spare parts are available for practically every joint and organ. So what has happened to the equipment for the hospitalized patient?

I sit today in a hospital bed with a Gatch frame—but this one—mercifully and electrically—can be operated by the patient alone. When I consider the frequency with which I make slight adjustments for head and knee and then think of patients once having to call upon the nurse for such services, my heart bleeds for both of them. I love my hospital bed.

And there my praises cease. In my modern, air-conditioned, picture-windowed room stands that old familiar bedside stand, still backed against the wall. It now has three little drawers, but each one as inaccessible as the single one of the past. The towel rack is in the same old place, too, still sandwiched between table and wall, to ensure that the towel stays perpetually damp.

Now no one—sick or well, lying flat in bed or sitting up—can ever open those bedside drawers unless he is a contortionist. So the first thing the knowledgeable patient does is pull the stand forward and then turn it around so that the drawers face the bed. (Inevitably, on any brief absence of the patient from the room, someone will move the stand back to its original position: "It looks better that way." Care givers also like to tie the signal cord to a drawer handle so that each time the patient opens the drawer, a disembodied voice responds with, "Can I help you?")

But repositioning the stand still doesn't give access to the drawers: Those infernal half siderails, usually left up because that's where the bed controls are located, get in the way. Somehow you have to snake your arm through the rails to get at the drawers of the stand and then coax the desired object back through the interstices. And to lower the rails while in bed calls for another gymnastic feat: You have to lean out and over, risking life and limb—well, limb, anyway—to get at the control. All this for a tissue or a mint.

Now let's consider the over-the-bed table, which hasn't changed much through the years. It's undeniably functional: to hold the comb, lipstick, or meal tray. The adjustable height is another bonus, but with a catch: Different types of tables are raised or lowered in different ways. Some you crank; others you push a button; and still another kind you raise or lower by hand (provided you have Amazonian strength) until it clicks into the notch at the desired level. The trouble is that sometimes you only *think* you've fitted it into the notch; later it descends suddenly, usually with your meal tray on it.

I have now been promoted to a wheelchair—a nice, modern, plastic and chrome affair, unlike the wooden behemoths I once knew. I can maneuver it, lock and unlock its wheels, raise or lower the leg supports, flip the footrests up and down. Great! But what I cannot do is transport anything in it besides myself. My hands are busy rolling the wheels, and a lap is a precarious place to balance anything, especially a cup of coffee. There's got to be a better way—or attachment.

My pet abomination, though, is the plastic in which all hospital mattresses and pillows now come firmly enveloped. Today's nurses are great, I think, but even the most well-intentioned can do nothing about that ubiquitous plastic: The patient must just lie there and sweat. The damn stuff is slippery, too, so you wake in the night to find cheek pillowed on clammy plastic, the pillowcase having long ago slipped off to parts unknown. The solution? Bring your own pillow.

As I write this, the astronauts have just succeeded in knocking a chunk of ice off their spaceship to restore their toilet facilities. Perhaps they might now consider knocking some of the antediluvian ice off our so-called modern hospital equipment.

Why I'm Superstitious About Nurse's Curses*

GRETCHEN COURTRIGHT, R.N.

Unusual calm greeted the harried evening supervisor as she burst into the ICU. Nine sinus rhythms marched sedately across the monitor—not a jagged line in the bunch. The hiss of bellows was, for once, unbroken by the harsh sound of pressure alarms. Call bells were silent. The nurses sat quietly, catching up on their charting.

"I don't believe it. The rest of the house is having one crisis after another," the supervisor whispered with relief, as if she were afraid of breaking a spell. She dropped the report sheet on my desk and headed for the door, pausing just long enough to say, "I'm sure glad it's quiet in *here*."

At that, a chorus of groans arose from the staff. "Now you've done it," I added under my breath—for I knew that, unwittingly, she had laid a "nurse's curse" on us.

I wasn't at all surprised to hear a suspicious noise five minutes later. The occupant of the farthest cubicle was magically shedding his soft wrist restraints. By the time I reached his side, he had pulled out his arterial line. As I applied pressure to his spurting wrist, chaos broke out on the unit. Call bells buzzed, respirator alarms sounded for no apparent reason, and the resident appeared to ask which patient could be transferred to make room for a more critical one. And to think the supervisor's carelessly spoken words were responsible for the whole commotion!

Work-related Superstitions

I used to scoff at people who avoided black cats or refused to walk under ladders. My years as a nurse, however, have made me an on-the-job believer in superstition, particularly in what I call nurse's curses. The supervisor's innocent remark is a perfect example. It shows how one comment or action can trigger another—seemingly unrelated—event. Here are some examples:

• Indulge in a moment of tension-breaking laughter with co-workers, and the director of nursing will surely descend on your unit.

• Pull on those sterile gloves, and your nose instantly begins to itch.

• Start to give a patient a bed bath and the attending physician—long overdue for rounds—will arrive, along with an entourage of medical students, interns, and residents.

• Call a physician without the patient's chart, medication Kardex, patient Kardex, and laboratory values

*Published in RN May 1985, Vol 48(5), page 112. Copyright ©1985 Medical Economics Publishing, Montvale, N.J. Reprinted by permission.

right in front of you, and he's certain to ask a question that you can't answer.

• Witness a resident crossing his heart and promising with wide, innocent eyes *never* to do a certain thing again—and he will.

• Hear a doctor laugh at that "funny feeling" you have about his patient, and he's sure to get definite proof from you at 2 o'clock in the morning.

• Sign off a chart more than 30 minutes before the end of the shift, and the patient will—without fail—develop a problem that must be charted.

Just Another Coincidence

Every time I convince myself that nurse's curses are nonsense, something happens to undermine that conviction. Recently, our head nurse announced that we had to curtail our use of Chux because we were over-budget. No sooner had she finished speaking than the ER admitted two patients with active, uncontrolled GI bleeding to our unit.

Rationally, I *know* that our budget problems and the condition of those patients couldn't possibly be related. Could they?

If You're Married to a Nurse . . .*

GILLESPIE RICHARDS, R.N., B.A.

When my husband married me, pledging a troth seemed like a good idea. But I wasn't a nurse then. He had no idea of the indignities he'd suffer and the assessments he was yet to weather.

Twice he set limits: first, when I transferred the cat from anatomy class to our fridge and second, when he realized that while rhythmically massaging his hand I was really selecting a good vein. All the rest he has learned to accept gradually.

Looking back, I've found some helpful hints that might have made all our lives simpler. For example, the dog's heart rate is *supposed* to be irregular. As the vet told me, there is *no* need to call.

Another hint: Don't burden your children with a lot of technical words. Our five-year-old suffers occasionally from cold sores, which I made the mistake of calling by their real name. I guess I had it coming when, in church, he said in his too-loud voice, "Boy, does my herpes ever hurt!"

I should have known that there are really *three* techniques: sterile, aseptic, and benign septic. In the

last, my son sucks the scratch, covers it with a Kleenex pulled from the middle of the box (to ensure who-knows-what), and secures all this with lots of duct tape.

We've had a "marriage encounter" or two, but not in the usual sense of the words. Ours were hardly weekend getaways for meaningful interpersonal interaction. The one I recall most vividly resulted when both our intestinal tracts became happy homes for the *Giardia* family. *Giardia*, you recall, is a parasite that produces diarrhea, gas, cramps, and everything I don't like about the body from the waist down.

The medicine cured us of the acute episode, but my poor husband ceased all GI function: no stools, no flatus, and no appetite. His problem might seem quite personal and really none of my business, but I had done time on a GI floor where these assessments were big business.

I became frantic waiting for my husband to have a BM. After all, white bread plays a prominent role in his history, and he still likes to peel his apples. While reaching this new level in our life together, I reminded myself of the wife of one of my patients whose *only* concern after her husband's MI was his daily movement. She insisted that we call her with results. I thought also of an elderly man who, when asked about his bowel habits said, "Well, usually one each morning, but sometimes I have another at night, and those I just consider a gift from God."

Back to my own gift from God. By day six, I was beside myself. This man was going to have a stool, even if it meant I had to roll up my sleeve and . . . But nature did take its course and things started working "real well." They had to. He had had enough bran to empty a horse. All this after a few regrettable phone conversations with our long-suffering family doctor who had never heard of a Colace drip.

This is the same husband who agreed to see me through all things, without knowing what they might be. He's seen me through wifehood, motherhood, and nursehood—and still claims he'll stay around for old age. Even when I enter the Krebs cycle for the last time and experience lactic-acid buildup, I'll feel safe leaving my final dignity in his dear hands. For, however undignified we may become with one another, my code status is "no nonsense, only love." He knows I'll provide the same for him.

Hazardous
(to the) Waist*

TED ROBERTS

My wife, a dedicated follower of Florence Nightingale, claims her biggest nursing challenge is staying out of Room 423. There, Ms. Hardy not only has a cast halfway up her leg; she has a 10-pound box of dark chocolates right beside her bed.

"Have a scoop," she says to all the nurses. "No? Well then, take a few bananas. They'll just go bad." If that doesn't work, she thrusts a free certificate for dinner at the new Mexican restaurant (Casa de Muchas Calorías) right into any uniform pocket she can reach..

"It's a war out there," my wife tells me. "My floor is a smorgasbord. No sooner do I turn down a cheesecake offering in 412, when Ms. Barton in 410 tells me she won't make a full recovery unless I sample the white chocolate her nephew just brought her. Good thing the flowers aren't edible," admits my vulnerable wife, whose dimensions vary from those of a medium-size clipper ship in full sail to those of a dainty coastal schooner.

"Just yesterday," she says, "I was doing great. Our census was down, thereby reducing the inventory of nougat creams, banana bread, and doughnuts. I only had one wedge of pizza." (She didn't mention its thickness.)

"But then I stumbled upon Clarissa's farewell party." Five evening nurses means five casseroles, plus Ms. Barton's pineapple upside-down cake, brought in by a last-minute visitor.

Of course my wife is used to such temptation. And she knows that a little more padding here and there won't pop the ties that bind us. But it's tough on the new nurses. Soon-to-be-married Betty Sue appeals to her sister nurses for help. Her fiancé is into exposed clavicles; he mailed her a cookbook anonymously with recipes for carrot-and-bean-sprout salads shaped like pot roasts.

"I've got to squeeze into my wedding dress," Betty Sue moans. "If Ms. Lang—the one with the

Godiva chocolates—rings, please stand in for me. Don't let me hear the sweet song those chocolates sing."

Christina, who's been married so long that she'll mop up gravy with bread right in front of her husband, considers her own wedding dress but a dusty memento of her thin and unhappy youth. She's the first to volunteer for Ms. Lang.

You see, Christina's a locomotive that puffs up and down the hall a couple of dozen times a shift. Like weight lifters, steel workers, and coal miners, Christina needs her fuel. To such hard-laboring people, lettuce and tomatoes are hardly a main course; they're something you add to a roast beef sandwich. Besides, if you're planning to get Ms. Adderly in 425 out of bed and into the john, you'd better stoke up good.

Besides the goodies pushed by patients, there are all those farewell parties, baby showers, and impromptu binges that add their own special perils to the fourth floor. Actually, I don't worry about my graceful white clipper ship putting on too much sail. What bothers me is the one-way edibles traffic that moves from our kitchen straight to the hospital.

Many a night I come home to a kitchen that smells like a five-star French restaurant. A bean-and-burger casserole (my favorite) is bubbling on the stove, while a cheesecake does whatever it must do to ripen in the oven.

But just as the image of a golden slab of ambrosia has formed in my mind, my wife bustles by me, clutching the cheesy delight to her bosom.

"Where is that cake going?" I cry out in pain as she sets it gently on the back seat of her car.

"It's my supervisor's birthday and she just loves my cheesecake," she cheerfully replies. I should have known.

Of course the fourth-floor staff doesn't need a fancy reason to chow down. Somebody's leaving—somebody's coming. Finding a husband, losing a husband. When everyone's life has been uneventful for a while, they seize upon some obscure holiday to plan some huge feast.

"What is this?" I cry as she packs the car with delicacies, "National Starve Your Husband Week?" The question, I realize, is rhetorical. The only way I'll every score is to break a hip and wind up on my wife's very own fourth floor.

The Good, the Bad, and the Ugly*

DONNA HARRISON STAAB, M.S.N., B.S.N., R.N.

After 23 years as a registered nurse
A few observations in rhyming verse
15 of those years in continuing ed
Vivid memories flash through my head.

I was once turned in . . . to the state board no less
For teaching WITCHCRAFT . . . who would've
     guessed?
The subject was actually "Therapeutic Touch"
But for one poor nurse, it was just too much.
The system works . . . after careful review
One nurse was displeased . . . out of 92!
The incident left me a little scarred
I dreamt that the nurse had me feathered and tarred!

A few years ago, the month was September
We had a speaker I'll always remember.
For lunch I took her to the best place around
But the right mustard just couldn't be found.
She ordered a Reuben . . . not on rye but on wheat
No Dijon mustard so she wouldn't eat.
She sent back her coffee . . . made quite a scene
It wasn't fresh brewed, right from the bean.
At the afternoon break and this is no joke
We served tea and coffee . . . she demanded a coke.
We used paper cups, she had to have glass
If she comes again I think I'll pass.
She's still on the circuit in Kansas you see
But she's not doing any workshops for me.

A part of one workshop was so poorly done
I wrote apologies . . . to everyone.
The speakers were bored . . . and not well-prepared
I'd have sent everyone home if I dared.

We stayed to the end . . . then I wrote a letter
Wishing the workshop might have been better.
I invited them back . . . this time for free
They could pick any workshop they wanted to see.

I thought I'd seen everything . . . of course
     I was wrong
One of my speakers brought her dog along
I had to tell her . . . I remember her face
"We couldn't have dogs in a public place."
Seeing eye dogs, now of course they're okay
But nervous poodles must be taken away.
I tried tying him up to a stake in the yard
But the wind on the hill was blowing too hard
And yes, he was airborne for just a little bit,
My speaker looked out and just threw a fit.
We locked him in the car, what can I say
He barked and howled for the rest of the day.

But still I count my job as one of the best . . .
When we give Murphy's law a much needed rest
When the coffee's not cold and we don't run out
When the speaker knows what she's talking about
When all the objectives are actually met
And when the speakers don't bring any pets
When the nurses aren't sleepy from working all night
When the audiovisuals work just right
When everything clicks . . . and just seems to flow
Then you and I make a difference, I know.

My first 15 years in continuing ed
Enough has been written, enough has been said
If you get discouraged, just call . . . feel free
Cause most of the weird things have happened to me.

*Reprinted from Journal of Continuing Education in Nursing, ©1991;
22(2):49 with permission from Slack, Inc. Edited from the original.

Going Over the Hill*

CATHERINE M. NORRIS, R.N.

As a young nurse, I bemoaned the fact that older nurses did not stay current, active, flexible, aggressive, alert, and tuned-in. I decried the processes in which older colleagues participated that made them "go over the hill" years before their retirement. How could they let such a terrible thing happen to themselves?

At 22, I believed that all old grads of 30 (40 at the outside) were not as fast as they used to be, forgetful if not senile, out of contact with youth if not the world, and living in the past if not the previous century. Probably I even thought that learning, love, sex, strength, and power are finished by age 35.

Later, as an experienced nurse, I watched my colleagues strive valiantly to stay young looking, act as youthful as possible, and religiously keep up-to-date.

Both as a young nurse and as a middle-aged one, I was operating on false premises. People control their destinies, I thought. At some time they make a conscious decision to go over the hill or to fight the battles of staying professionally active.

Today, I see people as kidding themselves when they believe that living right, working right, and staying active will keep them alert, strong, and able to compete with the young Turks. They fantasize if they think that going over the hill is simply the lazy way out and that those who let it happen are somewhat less than they ought to be.

The pushing techniques are powerful, difficult to recognize, and more difficult to counter. Pushing can masquerade as respect, courtesy, and consideration. Or it can be a back-handed compliment that knocks you into the middle of the next decade but, because it compliments as well as slaps, is as hard to resist as the sweet blandishments.

Here's how it goes . . . At some point in your 40s you hear an occasional reference to how nursing must have been taught in "your day," or a reminder that you must have lots of memories about how nursing was practiced "back then" or even "in the good old days." Soon you notice that younger colleagues always rush to take the back seat in a car with only two doors, leaving the front, easily accessible seat for you.

If you *prefer* to sit back, as you're bound to with some drivers, you will find yourself in a wordless duel with some youngster, and likely to be outmaneuvered. She may weigh a ton, but she's very conscious that youth is more agile than age as she wedges herself into the seat you could have reached as smoothly as glass.

If you do win, the plumb cherub who loses will ask, "Can you manage?" Or with a cheery "let me help," she'll overwhelm you with a shove. As you land facing the rear window with one leg sprawled on the floor, your plight is proof that you are denying the diminution of your capacities.

God forbid that as you fall into the rear seat a garter should show! Her remark "I didn't know anyone wore garters anymore—I thought *everyone* wore panty-hose"—is a push that rates about 6 on a 10-point scale.

Giving up the back seat-front seat struggle just once sets a precedent—your first step over that hill. As you reach your lunch-time destination, the driver will stop at the front door of the restaurant and announce for all to hear that she wouldn't want you (the identified elder) to overdo. Or, if you choose a restaurant about a thousand feet from the building you're in, at least one of your colleagues will ask whether you won't get too tired walking so far.

At meetings that run overtime, someone is bound to ask, "Did we wear you out?" If there are stairs, younger colleagues always inquire, "Does it bother you to climb stairs?" or "Are you sure those stairs aren't too much for you?"

Crossing the street, a young colleague is unable to resist supporting your elbow. When you protest, she responds, "But we think you're special and we wouldn't want anything to happen to you." How can anyone deal with that without appearing to be an ungrateful wretch?

*Reprinted from Geriatric Nursing, ©1980; 1(1):40–41 with permission from Mosby Year Book.

People bring mail to your office, offer to return library books, ask if they can pick up something for you while they are shopping, and suggest other helpful services to a far greater extent than they used to.

It is thoughtful! It is kind! It is loving! But it propels its victims straight into the role structured for the elderly.

Once I arranged to do an independent study in a nursing home because requests for my consultation services came more and more in terms of older people's needs. After I'd been at the home for two weeks, the director of nursing said, "It's unusual to see a nurse your age interested in studying and learning."

Undoubtedly this was meant as a compliment. But when the speaker saw my shocked face, she backed off, saying, "I didn't mean to imply that you are old."

I heard not only "you are old," but the unspoken implication that middle-aged nurses are not motivated and do not learn.

I lead a full, satisfying professional life, but at nursing meetings or after an article of mine is published, someone nearly always says, "I see you are still keeping your finger in nursing!"

The rational comment would be "What are you doing these days?" or something to that effect. Reducing me to a finger is like saying that I'm over the hill except for a finger that is clinging to the good or vital side of the crest. What a fabulous picture this draws for the victim!

You can even get a pretty good shove in public. An invitation to speak at an American Nurses' Association convention is, for most invitees, a once-in-a-lifetime event. When I was so invited, I felt I had really made it. What a joyous ego trip—until I heard myself being introduced from the platform as "one nurse who has kept up-to-date."

The introducing nurse could not have been more than five years younger than I, but that's really not the point. The point here is a kind of blame by implication. One should take for granted that nurse scholars are up-to-date. To mention it as praise says that one does not expect it and is surprised.

The data I have presented relate only to the behavior of nurse colleagues. Students and young family members push, too, and more directly. Nurses are more subtle, acting on stereotypes but using all the nursing ploys to imply problems of maneuverability, lack of strength, easy fatigability, declining interest or motivation, and unwillingness or failing ability to learn and to maintain an alert, intelligent, knowledgeable approach to nursing.

That the process starts when one is barely 45 may have to do with the generation gap or with competition for upward movement. Does upward mobility depend on unseating present incumbents? Or maybe we are trapped in the male scientists' (including physicians) view of middle age. At a recent invitational research conference on the menopause, men generally defined middle age for women as 35 to 50 years and middle age for men as 55 to 65. This would make women old at 51, and may partly account for casting them into "old" roles.

Whatever the reason for all the subtle pushing over the hill, we need to be aware that we do it, how we do it, and how hard our methods are to combat. Let's recognize that middle age has its own problems. People do not need the ones manufactured by pushing.

I say, "Victims of the push, unite!" Learn to resist. Put up the good fight so that, as we climb the hill and approach the crest, we go at our own rate, playing our own drums, and not with a push or a shove.

The Last Nurse*

MELODY ALLISON, R.N., B.S.N.

Yes, you're the only RN today. Yes, you must still do all the physicals AND take charge.

We MUST cut costs.

If it's not documented, it's not done.

FIND a bed for this one.

Formaldehyde is safe. The fumes could not possibly have caused the swelling around your eyes.

I was afraid, but you made me feel better.

OF COURSE I want that done whether or not I write it on the order sheet.

We forgot the lead aprons. But don't worry, X rays are no more harmful than sunlight.

Routine chest X rays are mandatory for our preemployment physicals, regardless of what the CDC and USDHHS say. Sorry, that's our policy.

We're short. You'll have to come in on your day off. Yes, I know that makes eight days in a row.

You'll have to earn your mandatory continuing education credits on your own time from now on.

You MUST float to the cardiac step-down unit and take charge. It doesn't matter that you're from the nursery.

Don't confine yourself to written orders. Use your own judgment.

Don't practice medicine.

I'm sorry, but we've had two sick calls already. You MUST stay for the next shift.

While you're doing hematocrits, you MUST reuse your gloves unless you see blood on them. They are too expensive to use a new pair with each patient.

RNs are trained in all areas; therefore, they MUST float to all areas. That's hospital policy.

Good little girls get their reward in heaven.

AUTHOR INDEX

Alley, Pauline J., p. 150
Allison, Melody, p. 161
Armstrong, Nancy, p. 129
Ashmore, Jenny, p. 47
Beagle, Betty, p. 3
Blair, Roy, p. 5, p. 8, p. 11, p. 136
Braverman, Shirley J., p. 16
Buckley, Neal, p. 36
Carter, Michael A., p. 96
Cleland, Carol E., p. 132
Copp, Laurel Archer, p. 97
Cork, Ken, p. 17
Corr, Nancy, p. 57
Courtright, Gretchen, p. 154
Crabb, Joy, p. 57
Crawford, B. S., p. 65
Curry, Jill, p. 25, p. 32
Curtin, Leah L., p. 100, p. 103, p. 113
Dawson, Les, p. 124
DeWees, Virginia Moore, p. 91, p. 105, p. 133
Doyle, Jane Thompson, p. 115
Ensoll, Kerry, p. 4
Eynon, Laurie, p. 15
Gardner, Paul, p. 47
Gillette, Ethel, p. 13, p. 50
Goldberg, Joel H., p. 68
Goldensohn, Ellen, p. 75
Golightly, Suzanne, p. 134
Gore, Ellen, p. 37
Gott, Peter, p. 85
Grimes, Richard M., p. 76
Hengesbach, Carrie, p. 15
Hoffman, Robert S., p. 86
Huckaby, Cathleen, p. 118
Ingram, Mary R., p. 95
Janowski, Mary Jane, p. 151
Jarvis, Joan, p. 123
Jech, Arlene Orhon, p. 106
Jones, Sande, p. 51
Jordan, Karen M., p. 49, p. 69
Kent, Rachel, p. 4
Kerr, Avice H., p. 81
Khan, Delailah, p. 31
Kovalesky, Andrea, p. 55
Kron, Irving L., p. 79

Lankford, Thelma M., p. 131
LeMaire, Gail Schoen, p. 10
Lewis, Edith P., p. 153
Lorimor, Ronald J., p. 76
Mallison, Mary B., p. 141
Manchester Radical Nurses Group, p. 80
Mandell, Harvey N., p. 61
Mayo, Ross P., p. 28
Mihordin, Ronald J., p. 88
Milner, Connie, p. 21
Moore, Roy B., p. 120
Moore, Susan, p. 34, p. 53, p. 78
Norlander, Linda M., p. 54
Norris, Catherine M., p. 159
Parker, Judith K., p. 130
Pelton, Robert W., p. 42
Perry, Joan, p. 117
Plume, Angela, p. 99
Poole, Kathleen, p. 135
Radical Nurses Group, p. 7
Rhodes, Annette, p. 40
Richards, Gillespie, p. 149, p. 155
Richter, Pamela F., p. 20
Rinehart, Joan M., p. 145
Roberts, Ted, p. 156
Robinson, Tanya M. Sudia, p. 139
Rosenthal, Gloria, p. 109
Ross, Rene, p. 57
Ryan, William J., p. 121
Schrum, Marion M., p. 146
Schwarz, Thom, p. 63
Speitel, Rita, p. 57
Staab, Donna Harrison, p. 158
Stanton, G. K., p. 119
Swenson, Patty, p. 71
Telesco, Maria, p. 140
Tiger, Steven, p. 90
Vincenzi, Angela E., p. 107
Wabschall, Joan M., p. 102
Walker, Barbara Wyand, p. 84
Walker, Karen, p. 47
Weil, Carol, p. 19
Wheeler, F., p. 66
Wraight, Scott, p. 56
Wren, Sandra L., p. 125

BIBLIOGRAPHY

Are You Cut Out to Be a Nurse? Nursing Times 1987; 83(50):64–65.

A Consumer Speaks Out about Hospital Care. American Journal of Nursing 1976; 76(9):1443–1444.

A Cynic's View of the NHS. Senior Nurse 1987; 7(2):31.

Euro-Diseases. Nursing Times 1990; 86(34):42–43.

Injections–A Humble Task? Nursing Times 1981; 77(14):609.

Of Cabbages–And Eggs? Nursing Times 1982; 78(46):1959.

Reality Disorientation. Nursing Times 1981; 77(29):1269.

Barnum B: Losses and Laughter. Nursing and Health Care 1989; 10(2):59.

Barra JM: High Kicks in the ICU. RN 1986; 49(4):45–46.

Bawll ODD: The Quality of Nursing. American Journal of Nursing 1979; 79(1):196.

Berg A: The Reciprocal Natural Childbirth Index. Journal of Irreproducible Results 1991; 36(2):27.

Boyce KK: Deliver Us from Evil. RN 1982; 45(7):75–76, 78.

Brislen R: Divine Intervention? Nursing Times 1981; 77(5): 209–210.

Bynum JE: Will Visiting Hours Ever End? RN 1981; 44(4): 50–51.

Carter MA: Getting Our Act Together. Journal of Professional Nursing 1989; 5(4):175.

Carter MA: One Step Forward, One Step Back. Journal of Professional Nursing 1988; 4(6):396.

Cousteau V: How to Swim with Sharks: A Primer. American Journal of Nursing 1981; 81(10):1960.

Coyle R: Paper Sacks. Home Healthcare Nurse 1987; 5(4):56.

Crawford BS: Gown Tiers I Have Known. NatNews: British Journal of Theatre Nursing 1984; 21(12):20.

Curtin L: The Case of the Reluctant Role Model: From Health to Heresy. Nursing Management 1986; 17(7):7–8.

Curtin L: Selling Our Wares in a Not-so-open Market. Nursing Management 1986; 17(2):7–8.

Curtin L: Watch Your Language. Nursing Management 1987; 18(8):9–10.

Darling LAW: What to Do about Toxic Mentors. Journal of Nursing Administration 1985; 15(5):43–44.

De Angelis MM: Automatic Immunity. American Journal of Nursing 1978; 78(7):1278.

De Lauder L: Tears and Smiles in the ED. Point of View 1986; 23(3):21.

Dennis JL: How to Drive Doctors Crazy and Ease Them into Malpractice Suits. Postgraduate Medicine 1983; 73(6): 303–304.

Dock SE: The Relation of the Nurse to the Doctor and the Doctor to the Nurse. American Journal of Nursing 1917; 17(5):394–396.

Dowling F: The Business of Faith Healing. Nursing Times 1980; 76(19):820.

Downs FS: Writing Up–and Down. Nursing Research 1988; 37(4):195.

Duncan ML: Return of the Prodigal Nurse. RN 1975; 38(12): 28–31.

Dupont J: The Turning Point. Nursing 1978; 8(1):96.

Eccles AM: Using Humor to Relieve Stress. Point of View 1990; 27(1):8–9.

Edwards BS: Heart Sounds and One-liners. American Journal of Nursing 1989; 89(4):616.

Fahey PL: A Small-town Nurse Is Still a Nurse—And a Lot More. RN 1978; 41(5):60–61.

Felix C: Adventures in Nurseland. Imprint 1988; 35(3):76–77.

Fernandes RC: You Too Can Be a Difficult Patient. RN 1979; 42(5):55.

Fielder AL: I Remember When. . . Journal of Post Anesthesia Nursing 1988; 4(5):323.

Fischback R: "It Should Only Come to Pass . . ." Supervisor Nurse 1978; 9(12):32–33.

Francis B: Just Like Me. Journal of Nursing Care 1981; 14(12):14–15.

Freeman L: Nurse Versus Doctor. Surgery, Gynecology and Obstetrics 1927; 45(5):711–713.

Gillette E: Choice or Chance. Journal of Nursing Care 1980; 13(11):7.

Gillette E: Too Careful to Care. Journal of Nursing Care 1981; 14(10):4.

Glinsky J: Wednesdays Are Sunshine Days. Nursing Homes 1985; 34(3):33–35.

Goldberg JH: Across the OR Table. RN 1991; 54(2):48–51.

Hamessley ML: Cadets, March! American Journal of Nursing 1976; 76(2):243–244.

Harris P: Hospital Speak. Nursing Times 1988; 84(3):72.

Healey T: Odd Requests for Radiography. Journal of Irreproducible Results 1991; 36(5):22–23.

Hebing S: Humor. Advancing Clinical Care 1989; 4(4):43.

Henderson FC: If. NLN Publ 1990 #15-2344:23–25.

Hoffman RS: Hospital Utilization Review. Journal of Irreproducible Results 1991; 36(6):11.

Holcenberg JS: Academic Medicinemanship. Journal of Irreproducible Results 1989; 34(3):13.

Holmes G: The Doctor as the Nurse Knows Him. American Journal of Nursing 1907; 8(3):181–182.

Hribar KG: Nobody Ever Told Me: A Humorous Look at the Preparation of Critical Care Nurses. Critical Care Nurse 1990; 10(2):26–27.

Huttman B: Me? I'm Just Pushing Papers. RN 1980; 43(9):56–59.

Iles RL: A Dictionary of Pharmaceutical Research: Comments and Excerpts. Journal of Irreproducible Results 1984; 29(3):14–15.

Ingram MR: Some Skills I Thought I'd Never Need. RN 1985; 48(8):26–27.

Jackson C: NT Meets Nurse Nightshade. Nursing Times 1984; 80(49):43.

Jackson P: Why People Become Psychiatric Nurses. Nursing: the Journal of Clinical Practice, Education and Management 1990; 4(10):32–34.

Janowski MJ: One Dose of Sodium Spirit Diffuser. Journal of Emergency Nursing 1986; 12(5):334–336.

Jennings C: The Saga of the Older Student. Nursing 1985; 15(9):52–55.

Jobling D: Coffee Pots, Clean Sheets and a Star Patient. Nursing Times 1982; 78(36):1527.

Johnson HA: The Perfect Outpatient Operating Room. RN 1976; 39(11):OR-10.

Johnson LW: Homeostasis Conservation among Undergraduate Nursing Students. Nursing Research 1991; 40(2):118–119.

Jolley MJ: Why Do We Wear Uniforms? Nursing Times 1980; 76(22):961.

Jones IH: Over the Hill—And Far Away? Nursing Times 1980; 76(16):711.

Kelly LY: Contacts! Nursing Outlook 1980; 28(6):396.

Kerfoot KM, Buckwalter KC: On the Road Again. . . The Life of a Commuter. Nursing Success Today 1985; 2(10):16–19.

Knicely KH: Rx Humor. American Journal of Nursing 1970; 70(6):1261–1263.

Koss C: The Day of Thanksgiving. American Journal of Nursing 1977; 77(11):1876.

Kramer LA: The Audit and I. American Journal of Nursing 1976; 76(7):1139–1141.

Larson ML: Clockwork Poodle. Perspectives in Psychiatric Care 1972; 10(3):122.

LaRue C: The Wonderful Variety of Pill-Takers. RN 1976; 39(8):50–52.

Laska L: The Frivolous Medical Malpractice Case: A New Definition. Journal of Irreproducible Results 1987; 33(1):5–6.

Lassetter J: Educating Interns: All in a Day's Work. RN 1984; 47(4):85–86.

Laury GV: How to Win Accreditation (Without Really Trying). Hospital Practice 1983; 18(8):76–77, 81–82, 85.

Lindsay G: Roast Pheasant and Raspberries? Nursing Times 1980; 76(3):131.

Lloyd M: Baseball Lessons for Nurses. Nursing Outlook 1984; 32(4):200–203.

Macfie CE: Spots of Trouble. Nursing Times 1981; 77(4):171.

Mackay K: Test Yourself . . . And Everybody Else. American Journal of Nursing 1977; 77(2):342.

Mallison MB: Exactly Like a Nurse. American Journal of Nursing 1988; 88(5):629.

Mallison MB: The (Health Care) Reckoning. American Journal of Nursing 1988; 88(9):1165.

Mallison MB: To the New Interns on July 1. American Journal of Nursing 1989; 89(6):791.

Malone RE: The Harmonics of Nursing. American Journal of Nursing 1988; 88(1):144.

Maxted P: Breastaurant Guide. Nursing Times 1980; 76(45):1987.

Mazzella A: Are Nurses Professionals or Patsies? RN 1986; 49(6):62, 65.

Metten A: Locked in the Lavatory. Nursing Times 1980; 76(32):1413.

Metten A: Self-help. Nursing Times 1981; 77(2):87.

Montgomery CL: The Hospital Employee as Patient. American Journal of Nursing 1987; 87(12):1687.

Moore P: A Sinister Tale. Nursing Times 1980; 76(27):1193.

Morrish M: So You Want a Cushy Job. American Journal of Nursing 1982; 82(11):1800.

Oleksij RC: Let Me Win the Lottery, Lord. RN 1978; 41(1):40–42.

Pelton RW: Funny Laws. American Journal of Nursing 1985; 85(12):1430.

Platzer H: Not the Multiple Choice Question Paper. Nursing Mirror NICG J 1984; 158(14):S15.

Plume A: Tarnished Ages. Nursing Times 1987; 83(33):22.

Plume A: The Young Ones. Nursing Times 1987; 83(39):24.

Psyche: Christmas Eve. Nursing Times 1981; 77(52):2246.

Psyche: Close Shave. Nursing Times 1982; 78(21):902.

Psyche: Pastry Surprise. Nursing Times 1981; 77(26):1136.

Psyche: Reality Disorientation. Nursing Times 1981; 77(29): 1269.

Rich V: English as She Is Doctored. Nursing Times 1981; 77(34):1481.

Richards G: The More Things Change . . . American Journal of Nursing 1986; 86(8):982.

Rosenthal G: Prepackaged. American Journal of Nursing 1979; 79(10):1892.

Rothman D: Layman's Handbook of Administration of Anesthesia. Journal of Irreproducible Results 1987; 33(2):9.

Rush B: How to Make a Lasting Impression on New Friends— An Epidemiological Approach. Canadian Journal of Public Health 1984; 75(1):98.

Schmitz K: Surviving Nursing School with Humor. Imprint 1989; 36(4):105–106, 109.

Schwartz D: Fruit, On the Tree of an Early Ambition. American Journal of Nursing 1979; 79(9):1664.

Scoggins JB: Communicate, Dammit! RN 1976; 39(3):38–41.

Scott D: What Price Education? Canadian Nurse 1975; 71(7):22–23.

Scrooge, Sister: The Ghost of Christmas Past. Nursing Mirror 1975; 141(26):48–49.

Sculthorpe P: Regrading the Solution. Nursing Times 1988; 84(40):48–49.

Sculthorpe P: When the Chips Are Down. Nursing Times 1987; 83(13):44–45.

Shaughnessy AF: It's Medspeak to Us, but Greek to Them. RN 1987; 50(12):28–29.

Smith-Hilton EA: Are You All at Sea When You Float? RN 1985; 48(11):65–67.

Snow K: Once Upon a Time . . . Today's OR Nurse 1984; 6(10):40.

Spooner B: Barring Accidents. Nursing Mirror 1985; 160(14): 34.

Stebbins LR: Just Another Day in the Emergency Department. Journal of Emergency Nursing 1987; 13(6):390–391.

Steidl SN: Is There a Nurse in the Neighborhood? Canadian Nurse 1976; 72(7):35.

Steven D: Lump It or Like It. Nursing Times 1992; 88(27):30.

Stevens CB: The Other Side of the Bed. Nursing 1980; 10(1): 104.

Sutherland S: Trading Places. Nursing Times 1989; 85(2):34.

Swaffield L: The Nightingale File. Nursing Times 1984; 80(51): 40–43.

Take-Out T, Put-In V: A Case History from the Hospital for Acrobatic Pathology. Journal of Irreproducible Results 1972; 19(2):18–19.

Tanner NR: Absence Therapy: Killing Two Birds with One Stone. Journal of Irreproducible Results 1990; 35(2):22.

Taylor JB: By Any Other Name. Nursing Times 1984; 80(1): 55.

Taylor JB: Epistles. Nursing Times 1982; 78(16):683.

Taylor JB: Honourable Spade. Nursing Times 1981; 77(37): 1605.

Taylor JB: Turncoat: Profundities over the Bedpans. Nursing Times 1980; 76(40):1759.

Taylor JL: One Nurse's Baptism of Fire—And Water. RN 1976; 39(1):42–43.

Terry JS: A Proposal for New Careers in Health Care. Perspectives in Biology and Medicine 1984; 28(1):35–39.

Thomas NP: Funny Things Happen on the Way to Becoming a Nurse. RN 1975; 38(4):46–47.

Turner P: Beware: Mum under Training. Nursing Times 1990; 86(34):33.

Ward MF: This Shrinking Life. Nursing Times 1981; 77(13): 546.

West N: Wake Up, Helen, It's Over. Journal of Post Anesthesia Nursing 1989; 4(5):356–357.

Whanger B: A Letter Home That I'll Probably Never Write or, Look What I Learned in Nursing School This Year. American Journal of Nursing 1978; 78(5):948.

Wheeler F: Gown Wearers I Have Known. NatNews: British Journal of Theatre Nursing 1985; 22(3):10.

White A: Strangers in the Night. Nursing Times 1984; 80(51): 52–53.

White D: Trauma—But for Whom? NATNews 1985; 22(9): 15–16.

Whiteside R: Six Chiles, P.R.N. Nursing 1983; 13(5):144.

Williams S: Comeback. Nursing 1979; 9(1):120.

Wood J: But, Would You Want Your Daughter to Become a Nurse? Part One. Canadian Nurse 1981; 77(9):26–30.

Wood J: But, Would You Want Your Daughter to Become a Nurse? Part Two. Canadian Nurse 1981; 77(10):18–21.

Zuck D: The Violet Catastrophe, Or Point Four of a Nurse. Journal of Irreproducible Results 1985; 30(2):2.